THE COMPLETE CARE OF

BABY ANIMALS

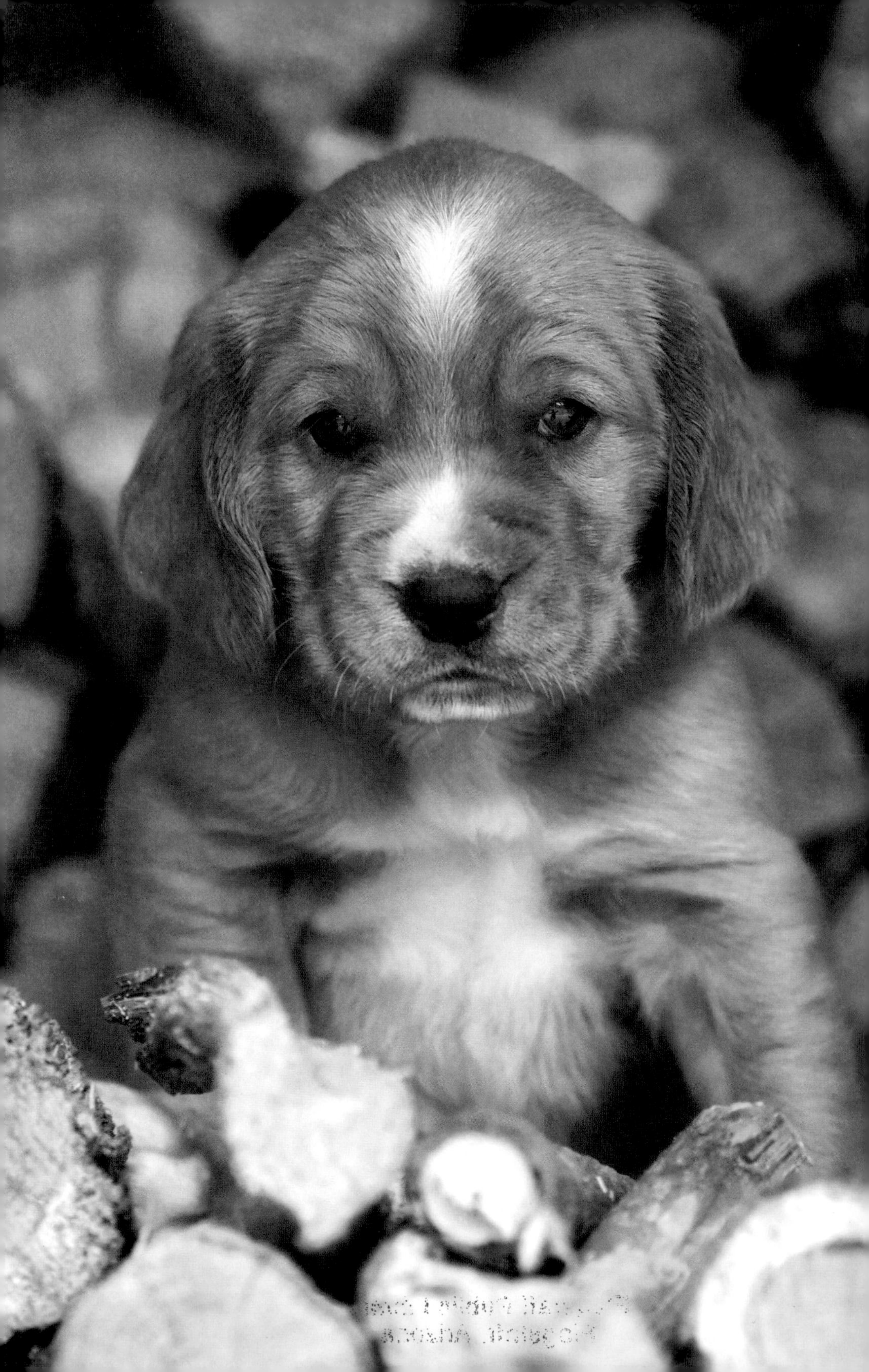

THE COMPLETE CARE OF

BABY ANIMALS

Expert Advice on Raising Orphaned, Adopted, or Newly Bought Kittens, Puppies, Foals, Lambs, Chicks, and More

BY *C. E. Spaulding, D.V.M.,* AND *Jackie Clay*

Skyhorse Publishing

Skyhorse Publishing books may be purchased in bulk at special discounts
for sales promotion, corporate gifts, fund-raising, or educational
purposes. Special editions can also be created to specifications. For
details, contact the Special Sales Department, Skyhorse Publishing, 307
West 36th Street, 11th Floor, New York, NY 10018 or
info@skyhorsepublishing.com.

Skyhorse® and Skyhorse Publishing® are registered trademarks of
Skyhorse Publishing, Inc.®, a Delaware corporation.

www.skyhorsepublishing.com

10 9 8 7 6 5 4 3 2 1

Library of Congress Cataloging-in-Publication Data is available on file.
ISBN: 978-1-61608-288-8

Printed in China

To all the special babies in our past and
future, the ones for whom this book was
written.

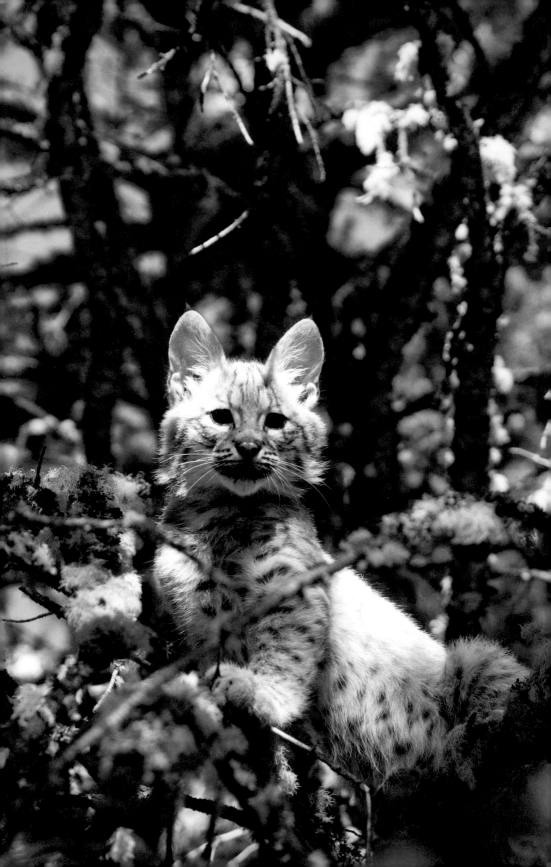

Contents

section 4

First Aid and Follow-Up Care of Wounds

section 5

Exotic Babies

section 6

Appendix

Introduction

IT WAS 3:00 AM when we became aware that the phone was ringing. I poked Bill in the ribs, while fighting the usual panic. At that hour no one calls socially, and it is usually an emergency. I listened to a groggy "Dr. Spaulding speaking," and tried to figure out, by hearing the one side of the conversation, what was going on.

In a minute Bill hung up the phone. A foal had been born that evening and the owner had just found the mare dead in the stall. He wondered if we would take the foal to raise—if not, he would "knock it in the head." At our house, saying no in such a case is unheard of. So, we got dressed. While I was thawing out some frozen colostrum (ko-ló-strum), the protective and nutrition-rich first milk reserved from a mare of our own, Bill got the coffee started. Then we sat down to wait for the new addition to be delivered, and we talked about some of our past animal babies.

There have been a lot of them, and there will be a lot more!

The smallest of the babies we adopted were two naked, blind, newborn jumping mice. We found these, along with a lumpy black snake (indicating the final resting place of the babies' mother and other members of the family) near a nest in a hollow log. The mice were about the size of large beans. With no electricity at our cabin and with tiny babies that needed the warmth of an incubator, we had to make do. They were popped into a pint jar, along with a handful of cotton for a nest. A few holes were punched in the top, and the small jar was suspended in a gallon jar half-full of warm water. The mice would be warm enough.

Then there was the problem of feeding them. Even we don't carry a complete line of baby animal equipment into the woods! And, even if we did, very tiny mice cannot suck from a doll bottle. Finally, we discovered a piece of absorbent string, which we kept soaked in warm

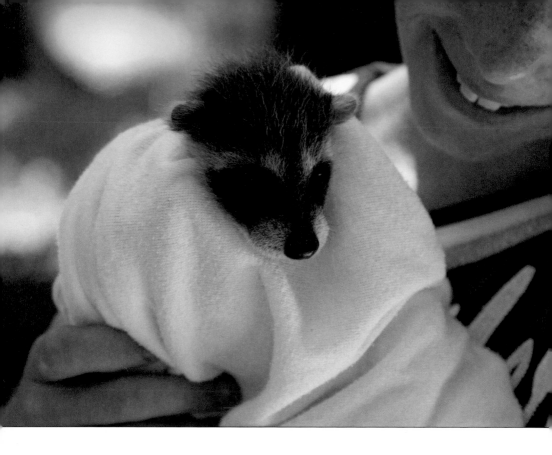

milk. It acted as a wick, and the babies soon learned where their new "mama" was, and "nursed" about every 20 minutes. The milk had to be changed every three hours to keep it fresh. But it worked! Soon they had a fine coat of fur and their eyes were open. It wasn't long before they would hop into a cupped hand and beg for treats. It was truly survival on a string!

The Grebe
in the Bathtub

AND THERE WAS Horace the grebe. He was a very late hatch and could not migrate when winter came on. The local game warden brought him to us, along with a permit, asking that we care for him. Grebes were quite rare in our area—so rare in fact that we had never seen one, and hardly even knew what one was! Horace's first home was a bushel basket in the kitchen. About all he did for a week was cuss and gulp down small minnows. And could he eat! I'd hate to be a mother grebe!

He grew and feathered out nicely. But, with size, he became discontented with the confines of the basket. He angrily hopped up and down, and eventually tipped it over. A big cardboard box was no better. Finally, a corner of the bathroom was made into a grebe "house." Remember that grebes, like a lot of other water birds, are messy house pets—and they show no inclination toward becoming housebroken! Both Horace and our family liked the new arrangement better, especially since the bathroom contained, of course, a bathtub. Soon that became a grebe pool. A lot of that winter was spent buying minnows from a local bait shop. Horace's daily ration of minnows cost $2.50! But, what the heck, how many people have a real, live grebe swimming in their bathtub?

Life with Dotty

WE WERE DRIVING to town one morning, thinking of anything but another orphan. On the highway, only a few blocks from the outskirts of town, I caught a glimpse of a little fawn on the shoulder of the road. She was alone. After a quick (and illegal!) U-turn, we pulled off onto the shoulder to watch the fawn. Something was wrong. A week-old fawn does not just venture about without a watchful doe very close by.

The fawn bounded onto the highway and ran up and down, bleating frantically. She was nearly hit by a truck before we could reach her. Then, frightened, she ran off the highway and into a woven-wire fence. By then we could see that her hind legs had been torn. We chased her down, with passing cars slowing to watch the "crazy people." Our intention was to examine her wounds, then give her a boost over the fence so she would not be hit by a car.

We caught her and carried her up to our truck, amid terrified bleats and a thrashing of very sharp, tiny hooves. Upon restraining her on the seat, we could see that the wounds on her legs and hind quarters were bites, either from dogs or coyotes. But, because we were so close to town, we strongly suspected dogs.

About that time, the local police car pulled up. From the policeman we found out that a doe had just been killed by two dogs. They had chased her right into town! That explained the absence of the fawn's mother and the confusion of the fawn. And, it explained the bites on her legs.

So, Dotty, the white-tailed fawn, joined the crew at the farm. We put her in a box stall, without a window, as we have seen a tiny fawn try to leap through a window five feet from the floor! Her first feeding was quite a battle. It took three adults to give Dotty her first bottle. The only way we could restrain her safely was to have me straddle her in a prone position, while a neighbor held her hind feet still, and Bill her front feet. In this ungainly and unlikely position, Dotty took her first bottle. The second feeding only took Bill and me. We were kicked a few times, but we made it. The third feeding I managed by myself, after backing Dotty into a corner. I still had to straddle her, but she remained standing.

She was getting less frightened, so I put a little goat kid with her for company. Fawns need company to adjust to captivity or they often either attach themselves to a person—making release difficult—or remain flighty. At first, she was frightened of the kid but within two days, the two of them curled up together.

It was late fall, and we knew that we would have to keep Dotty over the winter. She was born in late August, nearly four months later than normal. Alone, she would never be able to survive a bad winter. So, as she grew, we taught her to nurse from the doe that was the mother of the kid she "roomed" with. The doe was patient and quickly adopted a slightly different daughter. Whenever I would call Rosie (the doe), Dotty would come flying, hoping for a milk snack!

Dotty lived in the barn with the goats all winter and the next spring. She was free to come and go whenever she pleased, right along with them. As the goats ranged farther on their pasture, Dotty would follow along, finally growing brave enough to examine the edge of the woods.

It had been very hard not to make a pet of Dotty. She was extra cute, not only in her mannerisms, but because she still remained a fawn into her second summer. Her spots didn't fade until that fall, in fact. We knew that for her to be happy, we would have to let her be free to follow her natural instincts. And, we knew that if we allowed ourselves to make a pet of her, she would live a short and tragic life in the wild. So, we watched her play, with that funny little snort that really sounded like a sneeze, and resisted temptations to pet and cuddle her. And we watched her make the transition from pet to wild thing.

Luckily, we have lived in places that were isolated and surrounded by woods and fields. The babies we raise to young adulthood can simply take their freedom when they feel ready to. They are not dumped, unprepared, into the wild. They simply melt into the woods.

First, Dotty would spend the day in the woods, always returning for her grain and the security of the barn in the night. But, then there was the day she did not come back. To make matters worse for us, we heard a coyote howling a few hundred feet from the barn. We spent a restless night, wondering if Dotty had been attacked and eaten while we lay helpless to save her.

But when we went out to the barn (very early that morning!) and called "Rosie," a smallish, graceful shape bounded out of some willows near the fence and Dotty was back, licking her nose and wagging her fluffy white tail. I'm afraid we gave her a bit too much grain that morning, but she never complained at all.

It was the beginning of her freedom. As she gained courage, she began spending more time away from the farm. When she was sighted, we would get reports from all the neighbors, who knew about Dotty by now. "We saw Dotty today. She was crossing the swamp onto the high island." "Dotty was on the road, playing. But she moved off when we got close."

Dotty would let us get within a hundred feet of her—no closer!— after she left for the last time. But she never again came to the barn. She now lives in the swampy area and woods around our farm, and we see her from time to time, grazing on the new seeding in the hay field. We are hoping she brings a fawn with her, as the clover sprouts this spring. Then we'll know she has made her return to wild life complete.

Since first publishing this book, let me tell you that Dotty did, indeed, present us with fawns. In fact, she had fawns and brought them to us for six years. They were usually twins, with an occasional single birth. She would come when I called and eat the grain I left for them, but she would never venture closer and her babies remained truly wild. She was a true success story of raising a baby wildling who returned gracefully to the wild to lead a long and productive natural life.

Wolfling, the Coyote Who Decided to Be a Dog

WOLFLING DIDN'T LIKE the wild life at all! Wolfie is a coyote who was given to us by a friend who raises skunks, ferrets, and coyotes. Ken brought us Wolfling when he was about three weeks old, along with a de-scented baby skunk we had wanted for a house-pet. (A skunk is one wild animal that adjusts extremely well to people and domestic life.) The woman who had been taking care of Ken's coyote pups was supposed to be bottle-raising the pups. As it turned out, she was just putting a pan of food out, and letting them try to eat. Wolfie was thin, weak, and depressed. He was small for his age and scarcely had his eyes open. He looked like a little werewolf, with his unkempt, grizzled, black puppy coat sticking out at all angles from his pointed face and tiny, beady eyes. So the name Wolf was tried, soon to be changed to a more endearing Wolfie or Wolfling.

He was tube-fed for three days, as he could not, or would not nurse from a bottle. The day after we got him, he exhibited a severe diarrhea. We quickly saw one reason he was so thin and depressed. Anti-diarrheal medicine was begun, and other necessary drugs were given. He spent a week in the incubator (which we had recently purchased from a human hospital for *our* crew of "babies"). After a week of discouragement, when we didn't know if Wolfie would make it or not, the diarrhea cleared up. He began to eat well, and to act like a puppy. Soon, Wolfling was the terror of the house. The only one who could get the better of him was the skunk, Odie (eau de cologne!). Odie would wrestle and bounce around with Wolfling until he got tired of it; then he would pounce on Wolfie's head, giving his ear a good pinch. Wolfie would screech, dash off, and quickly recover enough to pounce on our ankles the rest of the day—while Odie climbed onto the couch and burrowed under the covers for a nap.

When Wolfling got older, he was too rough for Odie, so we brought one of our Afghan puppies into the house to be a playmate for him. The two got along like brothers. Wolfie was smaller, but was the initiator of all roughhousing.

Wolfie never did get housebroken. Rather, we were trained to put him out before he had to "go." As long as he was put out often enough, he was respectable in the house. It wasn't that he knew he shouldn't go in the house but rather that outside he used all his "ammunition" in marking his territory and had nothing left when he came indoors.

As with most of our other wild babies, we let him come and go at will. We did have to watch the Afghan puppy, as we didn't want *him* to follow his outlaw "brother" into the wild. Finally came the day that Wolfling decided to be a "big coyote" and return to the wild. We didn't see a sign of him for three weeks. (Except that every time one of us accidentally left the barn door open at night, a chicken would turn up missing!)

Then, one night I was waiting up for Bill to come home from a call. It was warm out, so I opened the door. Through the screen wafted the odor of *skunk*, and nearby. I quickly closed the door, not wanting the house to absorb the odor. In five minutes, there was a terrific barking from the kennel dogs, and a pounding on the back door.

All I could think was that Bill had stepped on a skunk! I went to the door and opened it. I was almost knocked flat, both by Wolfling bolting through the door—and the smell that accompanied him! It was Wolfie that had run into the skunk, evidently trying to play with his old buddy Odie. Only this skunk was neither playful—nor descented!

That was Wolfling's last try at wild life. Every after that night, he refused to leave the yard.

We kept Wolfling in the house until he was eight months old. As his natural instincts grew stronger, he became harder to live with. He had no compunctions about tearing the trash bag open and strewing it around. We could live around that. We just kept the trash behind closed doors. He would bite if you tried to make him get off the couch so someone could sit there. We could live with that. We just moved another couch into the room.

But, when he jumped up on the dinner table and stood guarding a perfectly done beef roast, we decided that he needed to become a wild coyote. The next day, I packed up the Suburban with a canoe, supplies, and a tent and drove to the northern part of the Superior National Forest with Wolfling. We put the canoe on a small, remote lake, in a chain of little traveled rivers and lakes. None were particularly beautiful, and there weren't any sport fish to draw fishermen. A perfect spot to release a needs-to-be-wild coyote! We canoed all day, crossing beaver dams, and hauling the canoe over shallows. Finally, we found a nice open camp site and pitched camp. I fed Wolfling his supper and kept him on a chain all night; I didn't want him to panic and run off into the wilderness without preparation. The next morning, he was happy and curious so I let him roam freely. We hiked along the lakeshore and he enjoyed pouncing on mice and chasing abundant snowshoe hares. I caught a few small pike for supper and again fed Wolfling. But that night I did not chain him. I wondered if he would be there in the morning. He was. But he didn't show up until I was frying breakfast.

We did this for a week and he, like Dotty, slowly remained in the wild longer and longer. I was happy when he came back after a two day stay in the wilds with a full stomach and happy face. I was happier yet when he returned at the end of the week with a lady friend in tow! Of course, she did not approach camp, but lingered in the brush while Wolfling snooped about, ate a little dry dog food, then left with her. I left the next morning, leaving a little pile of dry dog food, just in case Wolfling got hungry. He was now a wild coyote and doing fine. His lady friend would help with his training from then on.

Along with these wild babies and many more, we have raised many domestic baby animals. Some were orphans, and others were sick babies that Bill had been called on to treat.

Henry, the Calf
in the Braces

ONE REMARKABLE BABY was a Hereford calf, named Henry. Bill received a routine (so we thought) call from a client to check a newborn calf that appeared weak. When he examined the calf, Bill knew that without a lot of human help, the calf would never live. Not only was it weak, but it also knuckled over on both front and hind feet and could not raise its head to nurse. Had the calf had another owner, he would have been doomed. Very few farmers can spend extra time or will spend extra money on one calf. Luckily, Henry's owners were a family that really cared about the animals they owned and thought only of saving Henry—no matter what.

So, Henry came home with Bill, tucked in the back of the van. The local blacksmith made a set of braces for Henry's legs, which enabled him to stand, unaided. Then came the daily chore of exercising both of Henry's legs and his neck. But we were not alone in our added work. The owners had to milk out the mother twice a day, to keep her in milk, so that when Henry came home (hopefully), he would have a good food source handy.

Now, if you have never milked a six-year-old range cow that has never been in a barn, let alone been milked by a human, you cannot fully appreciate the job they had. First they had to drive her up a chute, get a rope on her head, then tie one hind leg to the post. While she kicked, bawled, and lunged about, they milked her. And as if that weren't bad enough—they had never before milked a cow!

But they managed. And Henry grew stronger every day. After two weeks, his braces came off and his feet stayed in a normal position. His neck was still tilted down somewhat, but he could raise it enough to nurse. Henry still tottered a little when he walked, but we knew he'd get along better if he were with his mother. (And we felt sorry about the daily ordeal of his owners.)

Henry went back home. His mother gave a glad bawl when she smelled him through the fence and, as soon as Henry was in the pen, he ran to her in a zigzag fashion and began to nurse.

By now, Henry was a pet. He spent the summer wandering around the family's front yard, being fed goodies by "his" children. He only stayed with his mother long enough to suck, then back under the fence he crawled.

In the spring, it was nearly impossible to pick Henry out of the other steers his own age. He no longer crawled under the fence, but ran with the herd, evidently more content being a Hereford than trying to be a person.

She's the One
in Long Johns and
Earmuffs!

NOT ALL CALVES respond to treatment so fast, however. Bill received a call from another client. He had six beef calves with severe scours (diarrhea). Five of them were scouring, but still strong. But one was down, unable to rise. There she lay, looking like a dirty, moth-eaten rug—and about as alive. Of course, she came home with us immediately.

The calf never moved all the while she was in the van. She was in such bad shape that she was brought into the office and placed in a corner with a heat lamp for added warmth. She had a subnormal temperature (usually a sign that the animal is about to die). The next 24 hours were spent adjusting the calf's intravenous tube and needle, replacing the empty bottle of electrolytes (which was given to fight her severe dehydration), giving anti-diarrheal drugs, and cleaning up the foul-smelling mess that seemed to flow from her in an unending stream.

After 24 hours, the diarrhea stopped. But the calf was far from better. Sometimes you had to stare at her for five minutes to be able to tell if she was breathing or not. Many times we were sure she had died, then we'd see her faint breathing again. For three days, she never lifted her head off the blankets. But she had no more diarrhea and with the aid of the heat lamp, her temperature remained normal.

We began feeding our patient small amounts of goat milk frequently, via a stomach tube, but there was no response at all. This continued for another day. We were becoming very frustrated. By all common reasoning, she should either have died or gotten better by this time. But she remained in limbo.

Finally, Christmas morning, we woke up to a loud bawl from the office. I don't remember who got there first, but I do remember looking at our calf wide-eyed and licking her nose for the first time in a week! We just *knew* then that she would live!

She drank her morning feeding from a bottle capped with a lamb nipple. (We always use the lamb nipple on very weak calves, instead of the harder and larger calf nipple, as it is much easier for them to handle.) By the next morning, she was on her feet, butting hungrily for her breakfast. In a day's time, she was put out in a box stall in the barn and nursed hungrily on our old nurse cow. The scours never returned.

When we took her back to her owner, it was still the coldest part of the winter (our winters get *cold*, often -55°F at night), and we were worried about how our calf would handle range conditions. After all, she had been a house-calf. We told her owner that she had to be protected from the cold, but we were still a bit apprehensive. Bill went out to check her after she had been home two days. We need not have worried. Her owners left nothing to chance. There she was out on the range—complete with long Johns, a sweat shirt, and earmuffs!

A Christmas Baby

SOME BABIES RESPOND to good care right off the bat, others take a long time—unfortunately, some never do respond.

For six months, I had wanted a purebred Jersey heifer calf. In our area, this breed is very rare. There are one or two herds, but it is just about impossible to buy a heifer—or cow—from them. Bill knew how badly I wanted that calf, so when Christmastime came, there was a large card under the tree for me. On opening it, I about went wild. It read: "Jackie, a Jersey heifer has been born at the Stoltz farm, and you can pick it up December 30. Love Bill."

He had traded a lot of veterinary work to get that calf! I could hardly wait for that week to pass. The heifer had to stay where she was for that time so she could get three days of her mother's colostrum milk and get started off right. We didn't want to chance *her* getting sick!

Well, finally, we could bring her home. I remember walking down that long barn aisle, with beautiful Jersey cows on both sides, to a small pen bedded with bright, clean straw. And in one corner lay a calf that could have passed for a child's toy. It would have been impossible to have made her more beautiful. She was a light golden fawn color with a glistening black nose and a pair of huge, luminous brown eyes. I couldn't believe she was mine.

We carried her home, secure in one corner of Bill's van, where she would be sure to stay warm. Then, at home, we covered her with a blanket and carried her to a large box stall in the warmest part of the barn. (It was—35°F, so even the warmest part of any barn was about 40°F)

We had cows milking at the time, but decided to feed her goat milk, as it is much more digestible than cow milk. And we fed it from a bottle, to be sure she didn't get indigestion. (Calves fed from a pail often gulp their milk, causing indigestion and scours.)

She adjusted well to her change and, during the next week, she grew and became more frisky and playful. Needless to say, she also became a perfect pet.

Then, one morning, she had the scours. We immediately cut back on her milk and began dosing her with kaolin-pectin and antibiotics. She did not get better. We brought her into our bathroom so she would keep from becoming chilled. We put her on electrolytes. No change. The next morning, she was weak, but still tried to raise her head to be petted. We stayed with her all day and half the next night, trying to will life back into her, I guess. Nothing we did had any effect on her, and at 1:00 AM, she died.

That was three years ago, and I still get depressed, thinking about it again. But I know that it is part of raising animal babies. Sometimes, you do everything right, but some other force seems to be in control, and your efforts are in vain. You just never know. I guess that's why we try so hard. Any animal baby that is breathing has a chance, and it is up to people to help them to make the most of that chance.

...And One for the Little Girl Who Lives Down the Lane

EVEN SOME BABIES that *are not breathing* can be saved! Bill did a Caesarean section on a doe goat that was unable to deliver her kids normally, even with his assistance. While Bill began the surgery, I stood by with a pile of warm towels and a bushel basket, warmed with a heating pad, to receive the kids. The first kid burst forth into the room with a loud bleat. Bill did not even look at it, but held it out in my direction, while going back into the incision for the next kid with the other hand. I quickly dipped the umbilical stump in a jar of iodine to prevent infection, cleared the nose and face of mucus, gave the kid (a robust buckling) a good scrubbing off with a towel, and popped him into the basket. The second kid followed in like manner. It was also a healthy and very large buckling.

Bill was disappointed when I informed him of the sex of each kid. It seems that the owners had bred this doe to a very special, and now deceased buck, and wanted a doeling to be their daughter's 4-H project. The daughter had mowed lawns, babysat, cleaned chicken coops, and sold cookies, just to pay the $100 stud fee!

"There's one more in here," Bill exclaimed, with hope in his voice. And out slid a small, limp form, a third smaller in size than the other two kids. But, it did not flop, or even breathe.

I held it up by the hind legs, to drain the mouth and throat, giving it a couple of good smacks on the side with the flat of my hand. Still nothing.

"Let's see it," Bill said, still holding the uterus with one hand.

He cleaned out the throat with a finger, then put his mouth over the kid's nose and mouth, inflating the lungs.

"Check her heart," Bill commanded.

I did, feeling a slight, but steady beat. "Her?"

Bill nodded, continuing the mouth-to-mouth respiration. For five minutes this continued, until finally the tiny doe gave a kick, then bawled louder than either of her two brothers had. She drew first one deep breath, then another. I was in a daze. She would make it!

"Get me another glove," Bill said, breaking the trance. (He had handled the doeling and touched the table in the melee, and did not want to continue surgery with a possibly contaminated surgical glove.)

He continued the surgery, and soon the triplets were all dry and cozy in their basket, all demanding to be fed! You can imagine the little girl's delight when we called to say that her doe was doing fine, and that she now had the doeling she had wanted for longer than a year—plus two very fine bucklings!

Our Early-Morning Visitor Arrives

WE TALKED OF all these babies, and many more. Soon, the kennel dogs began to bark, signaling the arrival of a stranger. It was the farmer with the orphan foal! Every time a new baby arrives at our farm, there is a period of excitement. How is it? Is it in shock? Does it have diarrhea? Is it constipated? Does it have a normal temperature? Does it want to nurse? Has it nursed from its mother? Where is the best place to put it? (We've had babies in the bathtub, the bedroom, the office, in the barn, the milk room, the aisle—and even in our bed!)

The foal submitted to this quick, but thorough check. I suspect that the farmer felt as though he were getting the third degree at first! The foal was a colt (male). He was a mousy, grayish brown that could change to just about any color when he shed his baby fur. He seemed active and wanted something to eat. He sucked my sleeve, my ear, my elbow, and even the truck bumper.

I coaxed him into the horse barn, using his new bottle as bait. His wispy, wiry feeler whiskers never left the nipple, as though he had glued himself to it and would *not* let this new "mother" out of his sight!

He drank 12 ounces of the defrosted and rewarmed colostrum, butting the bottle and finally my stomach for more. But I knew that it was much better for me to return in two hours and give him another small feeding, than to risk indigestion by giving him a full tummy of colostrum.

The colostrum is the first milk given by the mother. It is necessary for giving the foal antibodies against disease at an early age. It also provides a laxative effect to remove the "stale" manure, which has accumulated during the 11-month stay in the uterus, from the colt's digestive tract. We always keep colostrum, stolen from newly foaled mares, in the freezer, "just in case." It is very hard to raise an orphaned foal without this colostrum.

The foal probably could have handled more than 12 ounces, but we always shortchange new babies. This is because we never know just how much they have nursed, or how long it has been since they *have* nursed. It is best to build up slowly to a certain level in feeding. This lets the digestive tract get used to functioning again, and also get used to a different colostrum.

The second feeding went very well, and I felt that he was ready for 14 ounces, as he was very hungry after the 12 ounces was gone. I searched the stall floor and found a black, gooey string of manure. (We never bed a new baby heavily so we can monitor the bowel movements closely.) I felt like rejoicing! He had passed the first test. Now to see what his bowels would be like after digesting food. I feel a bit strange sometimes checking here and there for manure, but it is the consistency of the manure that signals the first signs of trouble. I want to know *right now* if something is heading in the wrong direction—not when the baby is already in serious trouble!

The next feeding also went well, with a nice pile of yellowish, but formed, manure in the corner. I seldom stay in the stall with a new foal after I feed it, as the foal should still be hungry, and I have found that when a person stays with the hungry foal, it will quickly learn nasty habits, such as striking and biting. These habits make the foal a spoiled brat when it grows up. And, as it gains size, a dangerous one!

It is tempting to play with the foal. But foals tend to play rough when they grow larger, and it is unfair to them to get them used to play when they are small, then stop when they grow a little bigger.

Our new baby grew and prospered. In two weeks' time, he was graduated from the bottle and lamb nipple to his "own" nurse doe. With a little work, most goats can be trained to accept any kind of baby. We have found that foals do much better when allowed to nurse from a goat than on a bottle.

Pretty soon a new routine was established. The doe was called from the pen every two hours, and led onto a single milk stand. She was given a pound of grain to keep her happy, and the "monster" was released. It took exactly two feedings for him to learn where "dinner" was served. And thereafter, down the barn aisle he flew, into the milk room and right to his doe.

She would kick him until he quit being so rough, which soon trained him to grab the teat softly—instead of booting her up into the air in his excitement and exuberance. She was a doe that milked a gallon and a half a day, so she alone supplied the colt's needs for a two-week period. After that, another doe was enlisted. The two of them supplied exactly the amount of milk he needed, until he was weaned.

At two weeks, he began to nibble at a few pieces of Calf Manna that I put into his mouth after every feeding. At first, it was just a pacifier, giving him something to do after meals. But, finally, he actually began eating a little. At three weeks, he began nibbling a little hay.

Finally, one bright sunny and warm day, we lured him into the paddock, with its sturdy, safe pole fences. We fed him, then watched his reaction to the outdoors.

First he sniffed at the grass, blinked at the sun, then gave a terrific squeal. He exploded into the air, kicked his heels high, and tore off down along the fence. At the far end he stopped, sniffed the ground, and rolled luxuriously. Then he leaped to his feet and ran back, whickering to us.

Spring was here again, and our first "baby" of the spring wanted more to eat! I'm afraid I'm a little sentimental and cry at everything. Bill is not so free with his emotions, but I know I saw his eyes glistening before he turned back to the house.

Raising baby animals can take you through every emotion—from elation to terrible depression. I think that, in order to survive the extremes, a person must maintain the right attitude. You learn everything you can possibly learn about the baby you are about to raise. This means reading, researching, and asking people questions. Then you must sift through all that knowledge, and piece together the truth!

There are a lot of superstitions and many old wives' tales connected with baby animals. For instance, I'm sure you've all heard that "milk causes worms." It may cause diarrhea, but never worms.

In raising baby animals, you also must become at least a little informed on medications and first aid—just as you must when raising human babies.

And you must become very ingenious. It seems that I never have exactly what I want or need when I am presented with another animal baby in need. We sometimes wander through the whole house for hours, looking for just the right thing to "Mickey Mouse" a feeding apparatus or incubator for an infant with a special need!

When this book was first written, the laws and regulations regarding the possession of wildlife babies were much less stringent. We worked with our local game warden in our wildlife rehabilitation efforts; indeed, he often brought us wild babies who were orphaned (usually by road-killed mothers). Today, there are many wildlife rehabilitation centers, which must be licensed to operate. Unlicensed people are simply not allowed, by law, to "possess" wild animals, even to raise them to release back into the wild. Keep this in mind, as there are stiff fines and even possible jail time for possessing a wild baby animal or bird in your home without being licensed.

You must also realize that no matter how much you do know, or how hard you try—doing everything right—that some babies never survive. And you cannot take it too much to heart. Death happens. There is no changing that. If you have done your absolute best, you have to learn to live with occasional death, and be able to bounce back the next time someone drops off a little box at your door and says, "Will you take care of this baby?"

We feel that the elation of seeing a tiny, forlorn baby grow from a totally helpless infant to a sturdy and happy adult, able to get along with little human help, makes all the hours of hard work, sleepless nights, and periods of depression worthwhile.

In this book, we try to help you all we can, so that you have the best possible luck with your babies. We want many people to know what we have learned and to be able to pass this knowledge on to others. Perhaps one day, no one will "knock it in the head" anymore, but will try either to raise the baby himself, or to give it to a neighbor willing to raise it.

SECTION **1**

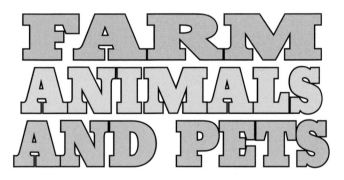

FARM ANIMALS AND PETS

Foals

ALTHOUGH THE FOAL is one of the hardest baby animals to raise by hand, excellent results can be seen, provided the owner has at least a little knowledge and a lot of patience. Always remember that even though the foal is quite large and sturdy looking at birth, in reality, he or she is quite delicate.

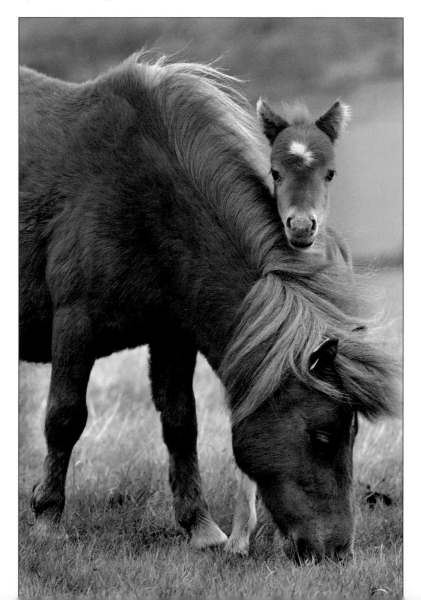

THE ORPHAN FOAL

On occasion, a mare will die during the foaling, or shortly thereafter. This presents special problems, in that the foal is deprived of the necessary colostrum, or first milk. This milk not only acts as a laxative, to get the foal's bowels working well, but it gives the foal immunity to many organisms that can cause serious trouble during the first week or two of life.

The best thing to do in such a case is to call around to several horse breeders and try to find a mare that has foaled, preferably the same day the foal you have was born. Then hand-milk enough from her to provide the foal's first feeding, which generally amounts to about six ounces. It is best if the owner of the mare will let the foal stay right there near the mare and let you milk the mare every two hours, taking what is necessary.

The mare's own foal will leave quite a bit of milk in the udder, as the new foal generally just snacks for a few seconds at a time. Some mares are very good about being hand-milked, but a few do kick. It is best to have someone distract the mare by gentle means, such as petting. If necessary, the person may have to use a twitch (a wooden handle with a small loop of chain slipped over the horse's upper lip and twisted tightly to get the horse's mind off the milking).

A mare is more difficult than a cow or goat to milk, as the teats are quite small, and the newly foaled mare's bag is often quite full. In milking a mare, do not try to pull the teats; instead, work the milk from the bag, down through the teat with thumb and forefinger on either side of the one half of the udder. The first few tries are apt to be frustrating, but don't give up. It will get easier. Don't bother trying to milk into a pail. It is too clumsy. An eight-ounce jar is much easier. Often, it will take a few strokes on the bag to stimulate milk letdown.

The foal should be given the colostrum milk as soon as possible after birth. The milk should be warmed if necessary, just so that it is not cool, but never hot. A pop bottle, fitted with a lamb nipple (available at most country drugstores or feed mills), works the best for feeding. A pail will not do. A foal will gulp the milk too fast and will usually get severe diarrhea in a short time.

It may take a little work to get the foal to suck the nipple, as it is built a lot differently from a mare's teat. The first feeding should be about six to eight ounces, with the same amount given every two hours, thereafter, day and night. If one feeding is skipped, the foal will be considerably weakened. If someone forgets to feed the foal at night, for example, that means two feedings are skipped and the foal will probably be severely weakened and is likely to die.

Soon after the first feeding, the foal should pass its first bit of manure. This is usually dark and quite gummy. This occurrence is very important, as many foals die from constipation, especially foals that are hand-raised. It is wise to use very little bedding the first week or so, in order that the foal's bowel movements can be watched very carefully. Bowel action is one good sign of how well the foal is doing.

It is wise to try to find a nurse mare, as it is a very tedious job to hand-raise a foal. After the foal has received a good deal of colostrum, call everyone you know who raises horses to see if any of them has just recently foaled and has lost the foal, or is an extremely heavy milker.

If such a mare is located and the owner is willing to let his mare raise the foal, it will be much easier than hand-raising the foal, provided the mare can be convinced that she should accept the foal. This can often be accomplished by rubbing Vicks or some other strong-smelling substance all over both foals, and also all over the mare's nose. Be sure to cover the foal's rump, as mares usually check the scent of their foals around the tail.

Tie the mare fairly short the first few times the orphan foal sucks, give her a good pail of grain, and bring the orphan in quietly, while the mare's own foal nurses. Do not upset the mare. In many cases, the mare will take to the foal after it nurses a few times. If she resists, a twitch on her nose or an injection of a tranquilizer will make her more cooperative. Take care that the foal does not get kicked, as this will discourage it from trying to nurse.

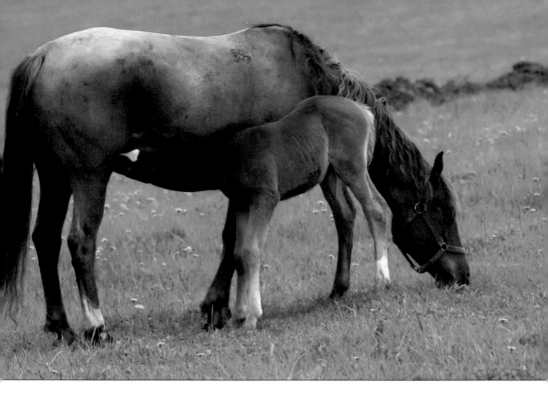

When a nurse mare is not available, the next best "mother" is a calm, fairly large doe goat. In most cases, with patient and persistent human help, the doe can be taught to stand still for the foal to nurse every two hours. At first the doe must be forcefully restrained. This is accomplished by having her tied on a two by three-foot platform which is elevated 30 inches from the ground. A regular milking stand works fine, as her head is in a stanchion then and only the hind legs must be held as the foal nurses. Care should be taken that the foal is not kicked, as it may be reluctant to nurse if it is kicked while trying to nurse. One person standing on either side of the doe can hold her still by leaning up against her body, while grasping a hind leg firmly. A little grain in a pail will also help to distract her.

It is best if the doe is not a first freshener (having had kids only once), but has had kids to nurse her several times, as she will accept this strange "child" much more readily.

The foal should nurse every two hours, but should *not* get full. It is well to know how much milk the doe does give, to know how much milk will empty the udder every two hours. Some does will give two gallons a day, where others will only give two cups. The doe that is to nurse a foal needs to give at least three quarts daily, and as the foal gets bigger, either a heavier milker will be needed, or a day mama and a night mama will be needed, as the foal's appetite increases.

The new foal will generally take from six to eight ounces and should not have much more. Frequent feedings are more important than big ones.

With the orphan foal, the nurse not only provides the needed milk, but also forms so close an attachment to the foal that it rivals mother love. The doe will lick the foal, talk to it, and provide company, all of which give the foal the will to live. A person *can* provide this companionship, provided he or she has the inclination, patience, understanding, and *time* to do it. Many people try to mother a foal, but end up injuring it. A foal cannot stand too much handling and excitement. This will cause so much stress that the foal often will die. Just nearness to a person is enough for a foal, with a little attention during feedings. Scratching the top of the rump or along the mane while the foal sucks the bottle is plenty of contact. Constant petting or allowing too many visitors the first week or two can be fatal.

Exercise is very important for the orphan foal. The foal follows its mother about in the pasture, making little side excursions on its own. Not only does this stimulate muscle tone and appetite, but it aids digestion and helps provide the will to live. A foal that does not receive enough exercise will soon become constipated and lethargic. Do not shut the foal up in a stall all day, trying to protect him from such things as drafts. Instead, allow the foal plenty of access to a grassy yard and encourage it to exercise as much as it likes, even if it is just walking about sniffing at strange objects.

THE REJECTED FOAL

In many ways, the rejected foal's needs are identical to those of the orphan. Colostrum, frequent feedings, a doe goat mama, if possible, and lots of time and love.

In most cases, a foal is rejected for two basic reasons: human interference and a sore udder. If at all possible, a person should be present at foaling time in case of trouble. But many times the person does more harm than good. An inexperienced, overanxious person often makes a mare so nervous that she is too overprotective of the foal for its own good. As the foal goes toward the mare's flank, looking for milk, the mare nickers at the foal and spins around to watch it. But at the same time she turns she is taking his supper away. Soon, she is extremely nervous and her bag is quite sore, due to all that pressure from the milk. Even if the person does get the mare to stand still, she often kicks at the foal as it tries to nurse, due to the pain of the tight udder.

A person who is present at foaling time should stay quietly out of the picture, stepping in only if there is trouble. If the placenta remains over the foal's head, if the foal is coming wrong or if the mare is in a bad position to deliver, a person in the stall is helpful, if he or she doesn't excite the mare. But, the person should remain there only long enough to correct the trouble, then leave the immediate area.

Some mares, especially first foal mares, have a hard, painful bag at foaling, and will kick or bite their foal as it tries to nurse. These mares can be given an injectable diuretic that will draw some of the fluid and hardness from the bag, relieving the pain. Also, if the mare is twitched or tranquilized, some of the milk can be taken from the bag by hand to help relieve the condition.

It is best to do everything possible to encourage the mare to accept the foal before deciding to hand-raise it, as the foal will have a much better chance with even a poor mother than it will by being hand-raised.

Within two week's time all but the very savage mare can be encouraged to mother her foal—that means she will be feeding her baby for at least four months so all the fooling around with that uncooperative mare suddenly becomes worthwhile!

THE INJURED FOAL THAT IS UNABLE TO NURSE

On occasion, a mare rejects a foal so savagely that she injures it, or the foal becomes injured soon after birth, or the foal is very weak at birth, and it is unable to nurse. These foals present multiple problems. Not only must the foal be fed, usually by bottle as it can seldom nurse a goat, but there is the injury to treat, when possible. Further, it must be decided whether or not to keep the mare milking so the foal can nurse as it improves. If the mare is to be kept milking, the formula for the foal is simple: mother's milk, warmed just slightly and given fresh.

If the mare is trying to mother the foal and not kicking at it, she can be kept right in the stall or pasture with the foal for company and encouragement. Be watchful that the mare does not paw at the foal, for this is natural as she encourages the foal to rise. But the pawing gets out of hand with a foal that is *unable* to rise, and serious injuries can result. Other horses should be kept away from the foal, as they will probably snoop about, possibly stepping on the foal and worrying the mare.

Often the decision is made to dry the mare up because she is difficult to milk, or because it is too much work. But keep in mind that any effort spent on the mare is only temporary, and worthwhile compared with bottle-feeding the foal for four months.

If a foal is weak at birth, it must be kept warm, even if the outside temperature is fairly warm (50° to 60°F), as many weak foals cannot raise their own body temperature to normal (about 100.5°F), and soon die. A blanket or two thrown over the foal will not help. The blankets keep in body heat, but do not produce heat (unless they are electric blankets!). A small stall, warmed by a heat lamp, seems to work best. In very cold weather, substitute the kitchen for a stall, and an electric blanket for the heat lamp.

When using any heat-producing apparatus, care must be taken to insure the foal's protection from both fire and electrocution.

The foal's temperature should be taken at every feeding to be sure it remains normal. A foal's normal temperature is about 99-101 degrees F. If the temperature rises above normal, reduce the heat. If it falls below normal, raise the temperature. This artificial heat must be maintained until the foal is active and can raise its own temperature when chilled.

In a few cases, the foal might be so weak as to lose its nursing instinct. Here, the foal should be tube-fed until it begins to suck. A fairly large, flexible French tube can be purchased from your veterinarian. If he doesn't have this, ask him for a discarded intravenous tube. This is either flexible plastic or rubber and will work nearly as well as the French tube which is rounded at the tip.

The tube is pushed slowly down the foal's throat, at least a foot-and-a-half. Be careful not to let it get cut by the back teeth if they are present. The milk is held in either a plastic intravenous bottle (if the intravenous set is used) or a plastic dish detergent bottle (if the French tube is used). The foal will swallow as the tube goes down. If the foal is not swallowing and coughs instead, the tube is in the wrong place. If milk is given under such circumstances, it will end up in the lung instead of the stomach. Pull out the tube and start again.

When the tube is in place, attach the bottle of milk. Hold it well above the foal's head and let it run. You will either have to squeeze gently on the bottle or add an air vent by poking a fairly large-gauge needle into the bottle, in order to have the milk run out of the bottle. The milk should not run too fast, or the foal will get cramps.

Constipation often proves to be a problem for injured or weak foals, usually due to the lack of exercise. Watch the foal very carefully to be sure it does have regular bowel movements. If in doubt, give an enema.

Whenever possible, encourage the foal to stand and move around with help. If a foal is down too long, it will probably die. Slinging a foal very seldom works out. The foal either fights the sling or just gives up and hangs there. Grabbing a flank with each hand and lifting will raise the hindquarters. With the hind legs braced, you can then grab under the forelegs and raise the other end. With a very weak foal, you may have to arrange the legs for best support. It seems that even allowing the foal to stand in this manner before every feeding will boost the foal's strength and help it to live.

If a foal is injured, your veterinarian should be called as soon as the injury is discovered. Many conditions that can be treated successfully if caught early, spell doom to a foal if left a day or two.

FORMULAS

Listed here are the milks, formulas or feed mixtures, in order of preference, which can be used to raise orphan foals:

— The dam's own milk, nursed or bottle-fed.

— Milk from a nurse mare.

— Goat milk, preferably nursed right from the doe.

— Cow milk mixed with lime water (ratio: one quart of milk to one pint of lime water). The lime water aids digestion.

Following cow milk and lime water closely is powdered milk replacer. One problem with the powdered milk replacers is that they do not always dissolve readily, so there are lumps of pure powder here and there in the bottle. Either the lumps plug the nipple or, if sucked through, can cause very serious digestive upsets that are sometimes fatal.

If you use a powdered milk replacer, use one formulated for foals, not for calves or lambs.

After six months, feed as you would any growing foal.

Bear in mind, when reading through the schedule below, that each foal is different. Some can get by with fewer and larger feedings, but some require small feedings given more frequently. The foal should gain weight steadily (use a scale or weight tape, a tape that gives pound equivalents for size, not your eye), should usually be hungry, and should be active and seem bright. Ribs should not jut out, but a healthy foal is not rounded with fat either.

FEEDING SCHEDULE: BIRTH TO SIX MONTHS

	Birth to 1 week	1 week to 2 months	2 to 4 months	4 to 6 months
Milk	6 to 8 ounces	8 to 12 ounces	12 to 16 ounces	16 ounces down to nothing
How often	every 2 hours	every 2 hours	every 3 hours	every 4 hours
Calf Manna	...	1/3 cup w/ milk	1/3 cup w/ milk	1 pound daily
Grain	...	...	1 pound daily (free choice)	free choice

SYMPTOMS OF TROUBLE— AND WHAT TO DO

DEHYDRATION CAUSED BY DIARRHEA

We would say that more foals die from dehydration, when being raised away from their dams, than from any other cause. Dehydration does not mean lack of milk—quite the contrary, in many cases. It is the lack of body fluids, salts, and chemicals. In foals, it is most commonly caused by diarrhea. Of course, people raising a foal without a mare want the foal to live and grow to a good size. Often, they feed the foal too much at a time, thinking that they are doing the best possible thing for the foal. After all, they are feeding the foal as much good milk as it wants! The overfeeding causes bowel upsets, which cause diarrhea. The diarrhea causes an inflamed bowel which provides a breeding ground for undesirable bacteria, resulting in more severe diarrhea. Finally, the foal becomes dehydrated, weak, and lethargic.

Diarrhea is less common in foals that nurse a mare or doe goat, as the foal snacks frequently, but does not take in large quantities at any one time. Both the mare and the doe goat will let the foal nurse for a short time, but then either move away or shove the foal away.

It is very important to choose a formula and then create a feeding schedule and stick to it very strictly. Any feed changes should be made *very* gradually.

With a bottle baby, diarrhea is the most important thing to watch for. *Never* disregard loose bowels. At the first sign of diarrhea, cut the milk allotment in half. If, after the two feedings, the bowels do not firm up, give three or four ounces of kaolin-pectin, repeated every two or three hours until the diarrhea stops. If the diarrhea persists (it shouldn't if caught early), replace the milk entirely with an oral electrolyte solution, available at nearly all drugstores or from your veterinarian.

Electrolytes are a mixture of body salts and chemicals, and the oral mixture contains a correct balance of electrolytes, plus a small amount of sugar to make the solution palatable. Milk is hard to digest if there is a bowel upset, and the electrolyte solution will soothe any irritation while the foal is being nourished and the electrolyte imbalance corrected. Continue giving the kaolin-pectin while using the electrolytes.

Generally, you will first notice the diarrhea when a bit of pasty stool clings to the tail. It is generally yellowish at first. When diarrhea is suspected, either remove all bedding to be sure, or place a makeshift diaper on the foal. This can easily be made up from an old towel or piece of bedsheet. After each bowel movement, wash the area around the tail. That way, if the tail later appears wet or soiled, you will know quickly if the diarrhea is gone, still present, or getting worse.

If the foal suddenly comes down with severe diarrhea, consult your veterinarian. This is nothing to fool around with. Many foals die from this within a day, unless they get intravenous electrolytes and correct antibiotic therapy.

Expect a slight loosening of bowel movements at about 7 to 10 days of age. This is the time that the mare experiences her foal heat (the first heat period after foaling). Even when foals are bottle-raised, they seem to have a little trouble with diarrhea during this period. Why? No one knows for sure, but it does happen!

CONSTIPATION

Constipation, right behind diarrhea, comes as a troublemaker for the hand-raised foal. Often the two of them will alternate in a vicious circle for a period of time. The foal may become constipated, often due to lack of exercise (remember that normally the day-old foal follows its mother in the pasture, dashing about and adventuring here and there). The hard fecal mass irritates the bowels until the mass passes, then diarrhea quickly follows.

Constipation is quite common in new, hand-raised foals and should be watched for very closely. It is harder to spot than diarrhea, as there is simply a lack of bowel movements. But if a foal goes several hours in a constipated state, it soon begins to absorb toxins from the bowel and becomes lethargic.

Again, when you suspect constipation, remove all bedding from the stall or diaper the foal. Encourage exercise. Often constipation can be cured by simply allowing the foal to run about with a person in a paddock or yard. Do not, however, chase the foal or harass it to the point of exhaustion!

If, after exercise and a feeding, the foal has not had a bowel movement, and if it acts a bit droopy or strains with its tail elevated, but produces nothing, give it four ounces of castor oil by mouth and a warm soapy enema (use a human enema bag and about a pint of water).

If the foal persistently gets constipated, give it slightly more milk per feeding and encourage plenty of exercise. It is not wise to give repeated doses of castor oil and frequent enemas. I cannot stress too much the importance of the exercise to help prevent constipation. Normally, the foal follows the dam for at least 6 hours per day. Most bottle-fed foals are housed in a barn and spend perhaps only 2 hours of the 24 walking about. Naturally the idle foal is apt to become constipated. If the condition is not corrected soon, the foal will die.

Besides the obvious lack of bowel movements, early signs of constipation include: slight lethargy, a noticeable lack of appetite, and a somewhat stumbling gait. If you are in doubt, treat the foal for constipation. Waiting until you get a definite diagnosis may result in the foal's death.

MILK ALLERGY

Although seldom seen, it is important to realize that some foals are allergic to certain milks. Sometimes it's cow's milk, a nurse mare's milk, or even the milk of the foal's own dam. This milk allergy usually shows up sometime during the first week of feeding. The general symptoms are: severe or persistent diarrhea, colic, and lethargy. Often, the owner, not realizing what is wrong, continues to feed the same milk, sometimes even force-feeding the foal.

This problem has been termed "acid milk," "sour milk," or "bad milk" by horsemen for generations. In a few cases, the problem *may* lie in mastitis (inflammation of the udder, often produced by an infection), which changes the milk and will cause trouble for the foal in many instances. You can check for this by squirting some milk onto a dark cloth to see if its consistency is normal—not thick, not watery. But, just as it happens among human babies, a certain foal is sometimes just plain allergic to its mother's milk or the milk it is being fed.

Where possible, consult a veterinarian who is experienced with horses to get an opinion as to whether or not the milk should be changed. Of course, it is hard on a foal to switch formulas, but it is still harder on the foal to continue feeding it a milk to which it is allergic.

VACCINATIONS

In the hustle and rush of feeding and tending the foal, some routine things are often forgotten. Vaccination is one of them. It is heartbreaking to finally get the foal raised, only to have it die from a preventable disease, such as tetanus or sleeping sickness. The foal should have an injection of tetanus toxoid as soon after birth as possible. Any foal, anywhere, can get a small puncture wound and come down with a fatal case of tetanus.

It is wise to contact a veterinarian to ask what other vaccinations he recommends, and at what age they should be given. Then mark the dates on a calendar that you use regularly, as months have a way of slipping past quickly. The reason that we suggest contacting the veterinarian is that he will know what diseases are common to young horses in *your* area. It is not wise simply to vaccinate the young foal for everything it is possible to vaccinate a horse for. Some diseases are seldom, if ever, seen in some parts of the country.

GENERAL CARE

The foal should receive as much out-of-doors exercise as possible during this growth period. Sunshine and green grass are a great help in raising a bottle baby.

It is also a good idea to begin halter breaking it at a very early age, as well as to teach it to hold each foot up to be picked out—a lesson in who is in charge. Foals raised away from their mothers have a tendency to become spoiled pets and, if they receive only attention and petting, they can soon become so nasty as to be actually dangerous. Do not be afraid to really slap the foal, should it nip or kick at you. If you watch a mare correct her foal, you will quickly see that no matter what you do (within reason) it will be less severe than the hard kick or bite "mama" delivers. And she won't have to repeat the admonition right away either!

Be sure the foal always has storm protection available, also shade from the sun. An easy way to do this is to just leave a shed door open so the foal can come in and out at will. Use a relatively small water container. A stock tank can be dangerous to a playful foal. Often they jump into it accidentally and are unable to get out. Some drown in such tanks. A three-gallon heavy rubber pail is ideal.

Try to keep the foal away from barbed wire fences. Foals do not see up close very well for the first few weeks, and they often get excited in play or fear. They can tear themselves badly on wire. A pole or rail fence is safer, especially if the fenced area is small.

Keep a mineralized salt block available to the foal. It will learn to lick the block at a very early age.

It is a good idea to have a fecal examination done by your veterinarian early in the orphan foal's life, as even a minor parasite infestation can sometimes make the difference in whether the foal grows well or is stunted, even whether it lives or dies. Keep in mind that few worms can be seen with the naked eye, so just because you don't see worms in the foal's manure, it doesn't mean that it is worm free.

Do *not* worm a foal "just in case" it might have worms. All worm medicine is toxic and should not be given a young foal unless it is certain worms of the type that the chosen wormer will kill are actually present. Not all wormers kill all worms. Some kill one or two families, others a broader spectrum, but no wormer is surefire on all types of internal parasites—no matter *what* some ads proclaim.

As the foal grows in size and begins eating more grain, always be sure to give the milk first, then the grain. If the dry grain is eaten first, the milk coming after can pack it down in the stomach and bowel, causing indigestion or a bowel impaction, which can be quite serious.

Calves

SOME CALVES ARE especially weak at birth, so weak that they are unable to stand or nurse. Sometimes these calves are small, premature, or have been in the birth canal too long. Some calves suffer from their dam's lack of feed, vitamin A, or poor health. (It is a very good idea to give a cow an injection of vitamin A, vitamin D, and vitamin E about once a week for a month prior to calving to help guard against her delivering weak or scouring calves.)

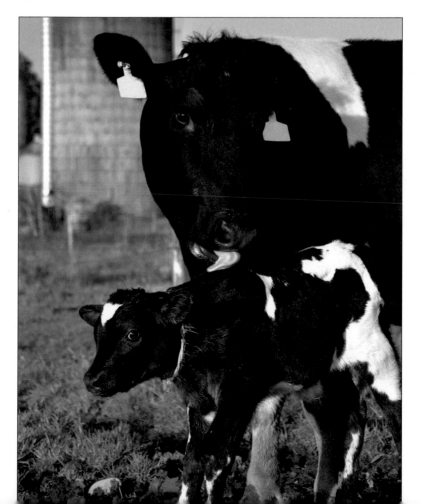

Any cow that is having any delay during calving (15 minutes or longer) should be examined. If the head and front legs are in place (like a diver), gentle, but firm downward traction should help the calf be born with little more delay. If the calf seems to be in an abnormal birth position, or if traction does not move the calf in the birth canal, quickly call the nearest veterinarian. Prolonged stays in the birth canal can and often do result in weak or dead calves being born.

A strong, healthy calf is on its feet within a half hour of birth, looking for its first meal—often in the wrong places, but still showing signs of hunger.

The weak calf is usually unable to rise, and can stand wobbly, only with help. Some such calves make feeble attempts to suck, but never do so with enough gusto to get a meal. Very few of these calves ever gain strength by themselves. Without help, they usually die within 24 hours of their birth.

The first thing to do upon finding a weak calf is to get a meal into it. *Never* pour milk down a calf's throat. This will only depress the calf, making it fight against drowning, and it can cause the death of a calf if milk droplets are inhaled into the lungs. If the calf absolutely will *not* suck, use a lightweight rubber or soft plastic tubing. An intravenous tube can often be promoted from your veterinarian, as many veterinarians use disposable intravenous sets which can easily be cleaned up for oral use. Do not use a hard hose or a tube over one-half inch in diameter or you will cause irritation, even damage to the throat.

If a special feeding tube or an intravenous tube is used, it will fit snugly over the tip of a syringe (minus needle), and often just a few snacks of about 30 cc of warm colostrum, milked from the mother, will perk up the weak calf until it can stand and nurse by itself. If you are using a 12-cc syringe, just detach the tube from the syringe, slowly push the tube down the calf's throat until it is well down past the mouth (be careful that the calf does not bite the tube, as they have very sharp back teeth), then attach the syringe full of milk and slowly discharge it into the calf. When the one syringe is empty, just detach the syringe, then refill it, and repeat until at least 30 cc have been given. Give no more than a quart every two hours, unless the calf is very large or is older than newborn. (Use a clean, plastic bottle of the type used to hold dishwasher liquid and tube instead of a syringe for larger feedings.)

If the calf should cough badly during any part of the process, withdraw the tube and try again in a few minutes. It is possible to get the tube into the wrong passageway and discharge the milk into the lung. This is not common. It happens when a person shoves the tube down without waiting for the calf to swallow.

If the weak calf has been born in cold weather, it is of great benefit to provide artificial heat, such as a heat lamp (or keep the calf in the kitchen), until the calf acts stronger. Even weak calves born in warm weather often have a subnormal temperature, and without artificial heat to raise their temperature to normal, the kidneys soon fail, and the calf dies. Keep taking the calf's temperature every two hours, until it acts stronger and has maintained a normal temperature for four hours by itself. A calf's normal temperature is about 101 to 102 degrees F.

Do not allow the weak calf to lie flat out on its side, as this discourages the calf and only weakens it further as it makes feeble attempts to rise. Instead, prop it into a natural position with slabs of hay or straw, changing its position at every feeding.

It is very important that the calf receive the mother's first milk (colostrum). The colostrum contains antibodies that protect the calf against diseases for the first few weeks of its life and it also gives the calf a good dose of vitamin A. This colostrum must be fed for at least three days. If the dam's colostrum is not available, use either fresh colostrum from another cow or frozen colostrum.

Once the weak calf can suck with some determination, allow it to nurse from the cow. Be right there for the first hour to make sure the cow accepts the calf and does not butt or kick at it. If the cow is not cooperative, place a figure eight around the hocks and, with her tied, hold the rope or twine and have a helper hold the calf in place to nurse. Usually, after a few tries, the cow will accept the calf, and all will be well.

It is best for the weak calf to nurse from the cow, as it will eat many small meals, gaining strength very quickly. If it is not possible to let the calf nurse, the calf should be fed every three hours at the rate of about one-and-one-half to two quarts, depending on the size of the calf, for about four days. Then you can slowly increase the feedings by about a pint a week per feeding.

THE SICK OR INJURED CALF

Sometimes a calf is injured shortly after birth or becomes sick and is unable to nurse. This situation must be noticed quickly and taken care of or the calf will starve. All newborn calves should be checked at least twice a day. They should appear bright, with large, shiny eyes, a damp, clean nose, and a clean tail. They should jump up as soon as they are approached and nurse often enough to keep the dam's udder nearly dry on at least one quarter. (New calves cannot drink all the milk from even one quarter of a good milk cow, but in a short time, they will take not only the milk from one quarter, but from at least two, or quite a bit from all four.)

If, all of a sudden the cow gives a lot more milk from the quarter the calf usually sucks, and the other quarters do not show any signs of having been nursed from, check the calf at once. Take its temperature. If it is over 102 °F, begin giving daily injections of a broad-spectrum antibiotic, or an antibiotic combination, such as pen-strep.

Check the tail, as new calves are often plagued with diarrhea called scours. The tail should not look wet or pasty. If it does, immediately give a good dose of kaolin-pectin, and cut the milk down. You can do this by milking the cow more than twice daily, so that the calf cannot get a lot of milk at one time. The kaolin-pectin should stop the scours, if given every two hours all day.

See if the calf walks normally. Sometimes a cow will accidentally step on a calf's leg, either breaking it or bruising it severely. If the calf drags a leg or carries it off the ground, call your veterinarian to examine the calf. If it is caught fairly early, a broken leg can usually be set on a young calf with little expense or trouble.

Any calf that is sick or injured may not feel like using the energy necessary to nurse. After missing a few meals, the calf is very much weaker, and then it certainly will not try to nurse. Without human help it will die within a day or two.

After the basic sickness or injury has been treated, measures must be taken to get the calf back to nursing. If the calf is not too dejected, the suck reflex is still present; however, the calf will not follow a cow around, nor will it raise its head and nurse. In such a case, the calf can usually be persuaded to suck from a bottle. It may be necessary to hold the calf's head in your lap, so you can guide its mouth toward the nipple.

If the calf has scoured, feed it lightly until the stool has returned to normal, or the scouring will get more severe.

When the calf is severely dejected and will not suck, you must use a stomach tube and bottle to feed it until the sucking reflex returns. Test the calf at each feeding to see if it will suck. As soon as it will suck, replace the stomach tube with the nipple.

When the calf again nurses well and strongly from the bottle, it is time to help it relearn to nurse. Give the cow a pail of grain and help the calf find the teat. There is seldom any problem from here, even when the calf has its leg in a cast.

BUYING THE SALE BARN CALF

People who do not have a cow or cannot afford to buy one often buy a calf at a local auction barn, because of the convenience and great choice, either to raise for beef or as a milk cow. Here, large numbers of young calves, along with a great number of other classes of livestock, are assembled on a weekly basis, to be auctioned off to the highest bidder. A buyer either pays so much a pound or so much a head (per animal). It becomes confusing, as sometimes some calves are sold by the head, and others of a similar size are sold by the pound, so a person must listen carefully. Also, there are a few things the auctioneer may mention quickly that might be wrong with a particular calf:

— A speck in the eye = blind, or nearly blind in an eye
— A little bump = umbilical hernia or navel ill
— Slow = calf acts sick
— Wet tail = severe scours

There are many other things that might be wrong, often particular to one geographical location. So it is a good idea to listen to that one auctioneer several times, and watch the calves carefully, if you are going to buy.

The sale barn is a risky place to buy a calf, so it is best to buy one elsewhere if you can. If you are going to buy at an auction barn, you had best know as much as possible about the calf before buying it.

HOW THE SALE BARN CALF GETS SICK

Why is the sale barn a risky place to buy a calf? Well, let's consider a few things:

— Some farmers know they will be selling through the sale ring, so they don't bother feeding the calf the necessary colostrum. Eighty percent of these calves die.
— Some farmers know they will be selling the calf, so they don't bother to feed it the day of the sale, and the calf goes 14 hours or more with nothing to eat.
— Some people just jam the calf into the trunk of their car or in the open back of their pickup truck on a cold day and drive 50 miles to the sale barn. Some of these calves are just born—not three days old!
— Some calves are sick before they ever leave home. The owner figures he's better off to sell the calf than lose it on the farm.
— The calves are all penned together, sick ones along with the well ones. Viruses and infections are traded with amazing speed.

—   The calves are not fed during the sale, and then face a long ride home, still hungry.
—   They are housed in an unfamiliar barn when brought home, adding to the severe stress they have already undergone.
—   The calves are fed a different milk or milk replacer than what they are used to, and maybe too much more than they are used to. This invites illness.

All these things happen at nearly every sale barn in the country.

Many of these calves are bought by inexperienced people who take very good care of them, but still they lose better than 60 percent of them! Why? Because a calf is very delicate, especially when it comes to the digestive tract. A day of severe scours can weaken a calf so badly that it will die. Few inexperienced people recognize this problem until it is too late to treat it effectively.

INCREASING THE CHANCES OF KEEPING A SALE BARN CALF ALIVE

Watchfulness is better than any form of later treatment. If a calf is to be purchased, *someone* must figure on spending at least two half-hour periods daily, watching the calf for the first two weeks. A person who knows what to watch for can quickly spot trouble and have the problem treated before it becomes serious.

The calf should be placed in a sparsely bedded stall for the first three weeks. Most people do just the opposite, thinking to make the calf as comfortable as possible. The problem is this: if the calf begins to drop loose stools in heavy bedding, the owner cannot spot it because the bedding gets trampled in with the manure, making it impossible to tell. Normal calf stools are orangish yellow and fairly pasty, not dark, fluid, or hard. The normal calf makes a lot of manure, which must be cleaned up twice daily to keep the calf clean and comfortable. Very little of this stool clings to the tail.

If the stools suddenly begin to get liquid or runny, cut the milk in half and give a good four-ounce dose of kaolin-pectin. This should be given every three hours until the stool returns to normal. If there is no sign of manure, but only foul-smelling wet spots, suspect severe scours and watch the calf until it is seen manuring. Usually, it will squirt out a very foul-smelling liquid stool. This quickly seeps away into the bedding, leaving little sign of its presence, other than the odor. This calf should receive no milk until the stool is normal, but should receive, instead, an electrolyte solution and kaolin-pectin.

It is a good idea for the new calf to receive a daily injection of tetracycline for a week after it has been brought home, to help kill any infection it might have picked up at the barn. Do not give medication past that period, unless instructed to do so by a veterinarian. Antibiotics can destroy necessary bacteria in the calf's digestive tract.

Calves under three weeks old are the ones most often killed by scours; then pneumonia becomes the number one killer. Any calf of three weeks or more should be watched for any sign of depression, such as not being very hungry at mealtime or not running in play. Very few calves with even severe pneumonia will cough or breathe hard at the onset of the disease. Lethargy is the first symptom. If the temperature is taken (this is done rectally with any thermometer), it will usually be above 103°F. A calf's normal temperature is 101° to 102°F. Often, the calf will run a temperature around 106°F, and just act a little "off."

This calf needs help immediately—not tomorrow! Tomorrow it may be dead, or at the point where permanent damage has been done to the lungs. Usually, a daily injection of a broad-spectrum antibiotic or combination of antibiotics (such as tetracycline or pen-strep) plus an injectable expectorant (used to get the calf to cough up the material in its lungs before they are scarred) for five days will clear up the trouble.

Continue taking the temperature after the first injections are given. The temperature should go down as the calf is treated. If it does not, consult with your veterinarian. A different antibiotic may be needed, and he will be able to tell you which one should work best, following the one you have been using. Some antibiotics fight with others; the result is that both are ineffective.

THE THREE-DAY-OLD CALF BOUGHT FROM A FARM

Rather than buy a calf at the sale barn, try to buy one from a local farm. This will cut down considerably on the stress to the calf, and give you a much better chance of raising the calf without sickness. You will be able to see how the calf is being cared for. (Is it in a clean area, fed from a cow or a clean bottle, for example?) You can also find out if the calf has been fed the vital colostrum for three days.

You will also be able to see its mother and possibly other relatives. This doesn't matter so much for a beef animal, but it is very important if the calf is a heifer and is going to be raised for a milk cow.

You can find out exactly what is being fed, and how much is being fed, so you can duplicate it at home for the first few days, at least. Then, if you want to make a change, it can be done very gradually so you don't upset the calf's digestive system.

When hay is fed to young calves, if possible it should be hay that has been in front of adult cattle, for they inoculate the hay with the

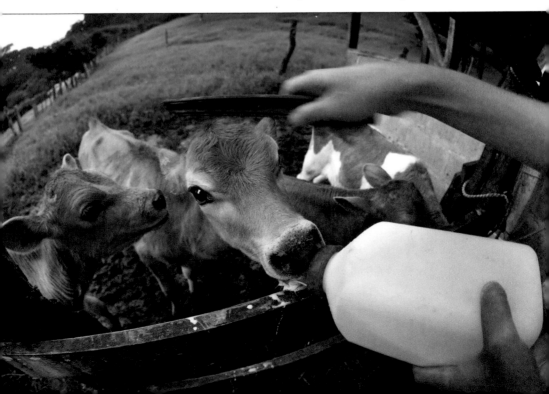

necessary rumen bacteria. It gives calves a much quicker start and avoids having calves with a potbellied look.

Be aware that the schedule below is flexible. The exact plan chosen will depend on the individual calf. If the calf looks too thin, you can slowly increase the amounts fed or the number of feedings. *Never increase feedings drastically or change formulas quickly.*

FEEDING SCHEDULE: BIRTH THROUGH WEANING

	Birth to 1 week	1 week to 2 months	2 to 4 months or weaning
Milk	1 quart	1 to 2 quarts	2 quarts
How often	3 times daily	2 times daily	2 times daily
Calf Manna	cup in hand	to 1 cup in pail	2 cups
Grain	...	free choice	free choice plus hay

SYMPTOMS OF TROUBLE— AND WHAT TO DO

DIARRHEA, THE #1 KILLER OF BABY CALVES

As we've said, diarrhea is *the* problem to watch for in new calves. This is true not only of the sale barn calf, but of any other calf on the farm. Calves born on the farm can get diarrhea, but it often clears itself up, provided the calf is nursing on a cow. Any calf with loose bowels should be watched very closely. At the first sign of watery or greyish stools, the calf should be taken away from its supply of milk and treated with kaolin-pectin, religiously every three hours.

Should the scours continue to an extent that feeding milk (which is actually irritating to the bowels) would be inadvisable, an electrolyte solution should be fed. Electrolytes are body salts and chemicals that are lost in severe diarrhea, along with fluids. The fluids can be replaced more easily than an electrolyte balance in the body. When this imbalance is not corrected, the calf cannot rehydrate and will die.

Often this is seen in a calf that is given a few "shots" (usually anti-biotics), but is also fed milk, even when force-feeding is necessary. The calf gets weaker and the scouring continues. More milk is fed. The calf begins to show a subnormal temperature and the scouring continues while it is fed still more milk. The calf dies and the owners are very frustrated. After all, they did everything (shots, force-feeding, and love), but the calf died anyway.

Irritating milk must not be fed to a calf with severe scours. Oral electrolyte solutions should be tried in its place. Do *not* combine the milk with the electrolyte solution. If the calf is very weak or if the scouring is severe, intravenous or intraperitoneal injections of sterile electrolyte solution must be given. Your veterinarian can supply inexpensive supplies for this and give instructions for their use. It is easier to learn by watching someone else the first time.

Basically, the intraperitoneal injection is given in this way:

1. Using a 3-inch by 16-gauge needle, an intravenous tube, and a 500 ml. bottle of sterile electrolyte solution, fit the needle on the correct end of the tube, and puncture the rubber stopper of the bottle with the other end. (A few older style intravenous outfits require that you *remove* the stopper, as one end of the rubber tube is flared to fit over the neck of the bottle.)

2. Invert the bottle. The solution should begin to run out the needle. All air bubbles should be run out of the tube, then the tube pinched off to stop the flow. (There is usually a special clamp attached to do this. If there is not, simply bend the tube back on itself or raise the needle higher than the bottle.)

3. Remove the needle.

4. Preferably, with a helper present, restrain the calf. The amount of restraint necessary depends on how sick the calf is.

5. Locate the site for the injection. This should be on the area in the triangle between the hip, last rib, and side. It also must be given on the calf's right side, as the rumen takes up a portion on the left.

6. The injection site should be cleaned well with soapy water or alcohol. Do not just pour it on, but scrub well in the direction the hair

grows. You cannot sterilize skin or hair, so you are just mechanically removing large numbers of bacteria.

7. Firmly and slowly shove the needle through the skin. (Don't go so slowly that the needle will not penetrate the skin. It is tough.)

8. Then continue pushing until it is in up to the hilt, with the hub of the needle resting against the skin.

9. Reattach the needle to the intravenous tube.

10. Unfasten the clamp to allow the fluid to slowly run into the calf. Do not go too fast or the calf will get abdominal cramps.

11. In small calves, it is best to give about 300 ml. at a time—no more—then repeat the dosage in three hours.

12. When the solution has been given, withdraw the needle and massage the area to help prevent leak-back and to ease any soreness.

It is also a good idea, when the calf has severe scours, to give antibiotics or sulfa to aid in fighting any infection present. Many calf-scour medications are on the market. Read labels. The calf should get more than an antibiotic to stop the scours. Kaolin-pectin works better than many drugs. In severe scours, the calf should be getting electrolytes, an anti-diarrheal (such as kaolin-pectin), and either an antibiotic, such as neomycin or tetracycline, or an intestinal sulfa or sulfa combination. Sulfamethazine and sulfamerazine are commonly used.

The calf with severe scours should have its temperature checked at least twice daily. If it falls below 101°F some artificial heat should be provided. A blanket thrown over the calf is not enough, as the calf is not producing enough body heat for the blanket to hold in. A heat lamp secured well above the calf, or some other form of safe, stationary heat is necessary. If the calf's temperature remains subnormal, the kidneys will fail, other body organs cease working, and the calf will die.

DIET TO HELP IN BOTH PREVENTING AND TREATING SCOURS

We have found that it is much harder to raise a healthy calf, using powdered calf milk replacers than milk. This seems to be in part, at least, that the powdered milk replacers are often not thoroughly mixed. If a person must use a powder, it works out much better if a gallon is mixed all at once, at least 12 hours before feeding it. This can be stored in a refrigerator, allowing *all* the powder to absorb the water. Hot water should be used, with the milk being very thoroughly mixed. Then it can be cooled down and stored. Before feeding, it should be brought to at least room temperature and *mixed thoroughly again.* Sometimes there are clumps of powder on the bottom of the pail that do not dissolve, even after standing for 12 hours! These clumps will give a calf indigestion *right now.* To be extra safe, some people run the finished milk through a cheesecloth, to be absolutely sure that there are no clumps of soggy powder. Of course, when many calves are being raised at one time, a few people can take these precautions, but when taken, they certainly pay off in good, healthy calves and fewer cases of the scours.

If the calf is being hand-raised, and you are using the powdered milk replacer, be sure to read the label and compare at least two brands. There are a few (generally cheaper) milk replacers that have little milk or milk products in them. These can just about starve the very young calf, due to the lack of digestibility or due to the ingredients themselves.

Although it is best to allow a calf to nurse on a cow, either its dam or a nurse cow, it is possible to raise the calf on cow milk, fed from a bottle or pail. Whenever possible, the calf under three weeks should be fed from a calf bottle, not nipple pail. The pail is just that—an open bucket with a nipple that sticks out of the lower side. The bottle is easier to keep clean and doesn't allow flies to crawl in. It also allows the calf to simulate nursing, instead of gulping the milk with its head downward, which is unnatural, but the way a calf is forced to drink from a pail.

When starting a calf on whole cow milk, you will have to feed it less than if the calf were nursing, as you will not be able to spend as much time feeding the calf as a cow does. In nature, the young calf sucks often, but only takes a pint to a quart at a feeding. This is easily digested, with no overload on the digestive tract. If you were to feed a three-day-old calf a gallon of milk, morning and night, all at once, it would probably scour in two day's time.

Next to nursing on a cow, the best substitute feed program is to have the calf nurse on a good producing milk goat. (If your does do not produce two quarts twice daily, use two does to feed one calf.) If the doe is placed in a stanchion, raised about two feet from the ground, the calf can easily be taught to nurse, and the doe to accept the calf.

If this method is, for some reason, unhandy, the calf can be bottle-fed goat milk, which is more digestible than cow milk. The reason for this is that the fat globules in goat milk are in smaller clumps, providing much more surface area for the digestion process to work on.

Should the calf come down with a slight case of the scours, you can eliminate the milk for two or three feedings, giving barley water in its place. Barley water is made by boiling half a pound of barley in a gallon of water. After it has boiled, reduce to a simmer, and cook until the barley is very tender. Drain off the barley (eat it yourself, or add to soup!) and give the water to the calf. It is very soothing to the digestive tract and provides some nutrition as well. This should be fed, about a pint at a time, every two hours.

WHEN TO CALL THE VETERINARIAN— AND WHAT TO TELL HIM

Any time your calf does not respond to your treatment and begins to show signs of weakness, such as a staggering gait or unwillingness to rise, call your veterinarian at once. Calves are quite delicate, and if they are allowed to get too far downhill, no veterinarian can save them.

Before you call your veterinarian, be prepared to tell him a few vital things:

1. What was the temperature of the calf before any antibiotics were given, and now?
2. What antibiotics were given, how much, and how often?
3. What other treatment has the calf received, and when?

4. Is the calf scouring? What do the stools look like?
5. How long has it been scouring?
6. What and how much do you feed the calf?
7. How old is the calf?

Such things as a continuous intravenous drip, cortisone injections, or different treatments are sometimes necessary, and your veterinarian, if called in time, might save a calf that would otherwise die.

VACCINATIONS

Call your local veterinarian to see what vaccinations he recommends for cattle in your area, as there are a few diseases that are common in some areas of the country that are not common in others. A few commonly occurring diseases that can be prevented by vaccination are leptospirosis, blackleg, infectious bovine rhinotracheitis, brucellosis (heifer calves only), and enterotoxemia.

GENERAL CARE

Generally speaking, calves are easy to raise, provided that one is alert to the problems that do plague calves, and treatment is given at once if any of them are noticed. Generally speaking, after calves are three weeks old, they are not bothered so much by scours, but they are open to different forms of pneumonia. Any lack of appetite or "tiredness" calls for an immediate check with the thermometer. If the temperature is over 102°F, call the veterinarian at once. Do not put it off or try to treat the calf yourself.

Calves should be outdoors on good clean pasture whenever the weather permits. All too often, calves are seen housed in dark barns, either in dirty pens or tied with a twine to the barn wall. These calves seldom grow well, are usually infested by lice and ringworm, have potbellies and bony backs.

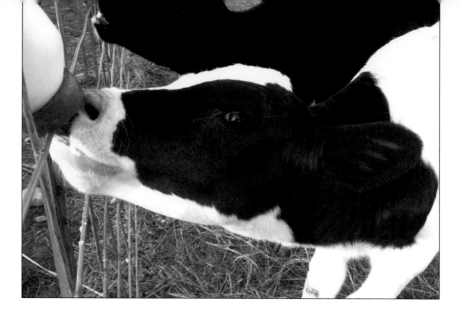

If the calf has access to even a small clean yard, he will do much better. Shelter is a must, but it is best if the calf can come and go at will. The shelter can be a small "dog house" type hutch or a stall in the barn having an outside door.

A weather-protected grain box, kept full until the calf is three or four months old, will help grow a big calf. This grain should be changed daily so the owner can tell just how much the calf consumes, and *what* it consumes. Calves tend to pick out the goodies and leave the nutritious stuff till last. Just like children. Keep tabs until the calf is eating three quarts morning and night.

A salt block is necessary. At first, the calf will lick very little salt, but as it grows it will need more salt. This block should be off the ground, preferably in the shelter so it does not get washed away by the rains.

If the calf is being raised to butcher and is a bull, it is best to castrate him at a young age. True, a bull gains faster than a steer, but with a steer, more gain is put on the meat-producing areas of the body, not just bone, head, and height. The safest way to have him castrated is to have a veterinarian castrate him with an emasculatome. This instrument crushes the cord and blood vessels going to the testicles, causing the testicles to shrink up and become useless. There is very little pain, no blood, and no chance of infection. The cost is also very minimal, especially if the calf is taken into the veterinary office.

Piglets

AMONG THE BABY animals on the farm that most commonly need human assistance is the baby pig. One reason for this is that a sow has, in many cases, a very large litter, not just one or two young. Even a single birth is a delicate matter, but when the process is repeated 15 times in birthing a single litter, the chances of problems also are multiplied.

Although there are few true "orphan piglets," there are frequent instances where a sow delivers more baby pigs than she has teats for them to feed on. Many times, a pig farmer will give one or two of the smaller piglets to a friend or neighbor to try to raise by hand, instead of just killing them.

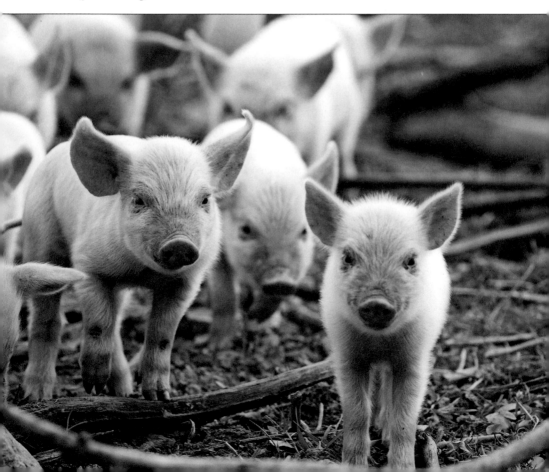

RAISING THE ORPHAN PIGLET

When at all possible, baby pigs should receive colostrum milk from the dam or another sow. The colostrum, the first milk the sow gives after the pigs are born, usually lasts three days. It is needed for its high nutritive value and laxative properties and to give the baby pigs antibodies against diseases. If it is impossible for you to give a baby pig a sow's colostrum, be sure it does receive colostrum from a cow or a goat, as it is the next best thing.

Baby pigs are most easily fed from a regular human baby bottle. However, their needle teeth (the sharp "tusks" are both top and bottom jaws) should be clipped soon after birth; otherwise, these teeth can quickly shred a rubber nipple. Even baby pigs left with the sow should have these teeth clipped, as the pigs are likely to cut up the sow's udder as well as their littermates. The best tool for clipping these teeth is a pair of ordinary side-cutters.

It is important never to overfeed the piglets you are raising. This can be tempting, as baby pigs are quite appealing, usually very hungry, and insistent. Feed them enough to make them almost full, but never so completely full that the abdomen pops out, round and hard. A pig that has eaten that much is almost certain to be stricken soon with a severe bout of diarrhea. A newborn pig needs between two and four ounces of milk, with egg yolk added. (We have had good luck with either whole goat milk or cow milk, one yolk per two cups of whole milk, beaten well.) The amount of milk to use will vary from pig to pig, so use common sense and vary as needed. The pig's skin should always feel snug, and its tummy should be round after a feeding, but should never look bulged and stuffed.

The baby pig should be fed every two hours during its first week at home, day and night. Even a few meals missed will result in a dead piglet.

Housing for the first two weeks should consist of a box about two feet wide by three feet long, and at least one-and-a-half feet deep. Baby pigs are very fastidious about their toilet habits. They will move as far as possible from their nest to answer the "call of nature," so cover one end of the box with newspaper or other absorbent material.

The piglet will also need a source of artificial heat for the first two to three weeks, free from outside drafts. A heat lamp is most often used, but a heating pad under a cookie tin which is, in turn, under the box, will also work well. The temperature in the nest area should be kept at 75° to 85 °F until the piglet is very active and can maintain its own body temperature. *Be sure the heat source is dependable and safe.* Many homes and barns have been burned to the ground due to an unsafe heat source. Do not have any cords or bulbs exposed to the piglet. It will play with whatever is available, safe or not!

If the baby pig has not had its navel dipped in iodine right after birth, it should be dipped as soon as it is brought home. Just pour some iodine into a widemouthed jar so it can be brought close to the animal for dipping the cord completely.

When the pig is four or five days old, give it an injection of iron dextran (150 to 200 mg.). Baby pigs are very prone to anemia, and early prevention certainly beats trying to treat a severely anemic baby pig.

The iron is given most easily by an intramuscular injection into the heavy muscle in the neck, which anyone can do safely.

Oral iron preparations, as given to human babies, may be added to the piglet's milk, as well.

After pigs are about a week old, they will start to nibble at a little solid feed. There are many commercial pig starter mixes available on the market, most containing about 21 percent protein. If a little of this is mixed with milk and given to the pig just before it is fed, soon it will be consuming quite a bit of solid feed, along with the milk from the bottle. Usually, by a week of age, the bottle can be dispensed with as the piglet will be learning to eat from a dish, and can be fed free choice both milk and mash.

Baby pigs' eating habits are a little messy, especially at first, so take special care to keep the box clean and dry. A damp, soiled box will soon result in a sick pig.

THE INJURED PIGLET— SPECIAL CARE

Often a sow will step on, or otherwise injure, one or more of her piglets. Many times it is just due to her very large size, compared to that of her litter. A 500-pound sow with sharp hooves can easily wound a 3-pound piglet very severely, quite by accident.

Injuries most often encountered with young pigs are either cuts and scratches, broken bones, or internal injuries. Cuts and scratches are easy to recognize; they are usually ugly and bloody. If these hurts are not serious, they can be dusted with a good antibiotic powder and the piglet can be replaced with its dam. (Be sure to use caution when grabbing that piglet for treatment. Mother sows are very protective of their young, and a few squeals from her baby can turn a pet sow into a man-eater!)

If the baby pig seems to need more than a dusting with an antibiotic powder, consult your veterinarian. Sometimes cuts are complicated by broken bones or more serious injuries that require some professional treatment as well as some further nursing at home. Broken bones are usually quite easily repaired by a veterinarian and, with continued nursing, the pig heals quickly. Broken limbs are usually fairly easy to detect: they flop, are not used, or drag. Swelling is common. Sometimes a person can see the ends of the broken bone pressing up against the inside of the skin.

Internal injuries are the most difficult to detect, and the hardest to treat successfully. This type of injury is often due to a sow's flopping down on a piglet or stepping on its abdomen. If the internal injury is of a mild nature, there may be a small amount of internal bleeding, complicated by pain and shock. In such a case, just removing the pig to a quiet, warmed box is often enough to bring about a quick "cure." Artificial heat is a "must," because a piglet in shock cannot warm itself enough to overcome the shock.

Severe internal injuries cause heavy internal bleeding and possibly the rupture of one or more internal organs. The treatment for this type of injury is difficult and costly.

Piglets with internal injuries often just act dumpy. On closer examination, the gums appear pale, and the piglet feels cold to the touch. Contact your veterinarian for a thorough examination and advice about treatment.

CARE OF THE RUNT PIGLET

Nearly every litter of pigs has one or more smaller piglets. In most cases, these quickly catch up with their larger brothers and sisters and weigh about the same at weaning. But sometimes there is a runt in the litter, a piglet that is considerably smaller than the others in the litter and does not grow well. A runt is often pushed away from the udder, bitten by its littermates, forced away from the warmest area in the nest and ignored by its mother. Seldom do these runts make enough gain to be raised profitably by a practical farmer. When raised alone, however, they often grow fairly well, and do pay off for the extra trouble it takes to raise them.

When possible, leave the runt with the mother until it is eating from a pan. At this time, it can be removed to a warm pen and special feeding can be started. A good pig starter mix, soaked in milk and fed fresh twice a day, usually gives the runt a quick "boost." It is a good idea to worm the runt piglet at three and five weeks of age, as some runt piglets are smaller due to a heavy parasite load. Use a mild wormer such as piperazine placed in the feed at this time.

Do not try to raise runt piglets that have twisted faces or humped backs. These piglets seldom live and, if they do, they just never seem to thrive.

If the runt piglet is in danger of starving due to being shoved away from the udder by its littermates, it is best to try to bottle-feed the runt until it can eat from a pan. (See the preceding section, "Raising the Orphan Piglet.")

FEEDING SCHEDULE: BIRTH THROUGH WEANING

	Birth to 2 weeks	2 to 4 weeks	4 to 12 weeks	12 weeks on
Milk	2 to 6 ounces	6 ounces plus mix with starter	1 quart mixed with starter	...
How often	every 2 hours	twice daily, keeping pan full	Twice daily, keeping pan full	...
Pig starter	...	1 cup plus	2 cups plus	...
Pig grower	...	...	...	full feed

SYMPTOMS OF TROUBLE—AND WHAT TO DO

DIARRHEA

One common problem in hand-raised piglets is diarrhea. Simple diarrhea is nothing to worry about; it occurs in nearly every baby pig that is hand-raised. Such things as feeding too much milk, a slight change in feed or formula, or excitement can cause it. When the irritant is removed, the stool again becomes normal.

It is when the diarrhea becomes severe or is longstanding that the intestinal tract becomes very irritated and often becomes infected with harmful bacteria. The diarrhea becomes worse, often watery, and the piglet will quickly dehydrate and weaken. It is very important to correct the situation before such a point is reached. Therefore, all diarrhea should be watched very closely and quickly treated if it should become necessary.

Should the piglet pass one extra soft stool, immediatey cut down severely on the amount of milk fed, until the stool again becomes normal. If simply cutting down the milk does not correct the problem, begin giving the piglet a tablespoonful of kaolin-pectin every two hours, before feeding. When this does not work (it usually does!), eliminate the milk and replace it with an electrolyte solution, such as is made for human babies with diarrhea. Continue giving the kaolinpectin and see your veterinarian for an antibiotic. This should be used for four or five days, even if the diarrhea subsides at once.

PNEUMONIA

Pneumonia is quite common in baby pigs and should be watched for. It is a mistake to think that because the piglets are well cared for and kept warm and dry, they cannot possibly get pneumonia. They can, and do!

The baby pig with pneumonia will quickly cease to be active and noisy. It seldom coughs, but does run a fever. The piglet's normal body temperature is 101° to 102.5°F, taken rectally. A piglet with pneumonia will have an elevated temperature, often 105°F or higher. So, on discovering an inactive piglet, take the temperature immediately.

Generally, when the pneumonia is discovered early, one or two daily injections of a good, broad-spectrum antibiotic such as oxytetracycline for four or five days brings about a quick cure.

If the pneumonia remains untreated for a day or so, the piglet's lungs quickly become scarred and permanent damage is done. If such a baby pig does live, it will be fighting for breath for the rest of its life. This will make weight gains slow. Also, times of stress, such as hot days or any exertion, will be very hard on the pig.

If you have doubts whether the piglet does indeed have pneumonia, by all means take it to your veterinarian for correct diagnosis.

MANGE

A common external parasite of the pig is the mange mite. These tiny mites are all but invisible to the naked eye, but burrow in the skin, causing intense itching. Mange is so common in pigs that large feedlots routinely spray the pigs for it.

Hand-raised pigs are very susceptible to mange, especially if they have had a rough time growing up. If the piglet begins to scrub its sides up and down on the box, furniture, or feed dish steadily, suspect mange. But be reasonable in deciding. *All* pigs scratch some, just from a plain itch, as humans do. A little scratching is normal. Constant scratching and rubbing is not normal. Spraying the piglet with rotenone or another insecticide recommended by your vet usually brings a quick end to the mites.

Often, it is necessary to spray the pig once a week for three weeks before all mites are dead and all unwanted scratching is halted.

INTERNAL PARASITES

We strongly advise that you have your veterinarian run a fecal examination on your pig at about six weeks, to determine if any worms or other intestinal parasites are present. Most pigs have worms to some extent, but the stressed, hand-raised piglet may suffer more from them.

A heavily parasitized piglet may have a rough, longish hair coat and be a bit potbellied, but appear thin along the back and hips. But it can appear perfectly normal—until it suddenly becomes very sick and dies.

A pig is not necessarily worm-free just because no worms are seen in its manure. Many times, no worms are found in the manure of a pig that is dying of a heavy parasite infestation. The veterinarian examines a bit of the manure under a microscope, looking for worm eggs and minute larvae which, if present in moderate numbers, can indicate a parasite problem *before* it harms the pig.

At the same time, the vet will also check for the oocysts (eggs) of a minute, one-celled protozoan parasite, *coccidium*. Coccidiosis is a very sneaky disease, as it shows few symptoms until the animal becomes so weakened by it that all at once it just dies. Often, infested animals have an intermittent diarrhea. Baby pigs are most frequently infected, especially those that are hand-raised.

The reason that hand-raised pigs are more susceptible is a combination of stress and a damp, manure-soiled box or pen. By the time a baby pig is six weeks old, it is likely to be a little "mess maker." We refer not so much to the manure, but to the fact that a normal baby pig is very active and playful, often spilling both food and water. This damp environment, along with possible fecal contamination of feed, can encourage the *coccidia* to become too abundant.

It is good to be aware of these problems, and to do everything possible to head them off. Keeping the piglet warm, clean and dry, and well-fed, but not overfed, will do much toward keeping it healthy as well. As the pig's size increases, be sure to increase the size of its pen. Pigs are naturally clean animals, using one corner of the pen for urination and defecation and sleeping and playing in the remainder. If their pen is kept clean and the manure not allowed to build up, pigs will never become soiled.

VACCINATIONS

There are a few vaccinations that are recommended for pigs. It is a good idea to contact the local veterinarian to see just which diseases are a problem in your particular area of the country, and which vaccinations he recommends.

A few common vaccinations for pigs are: hog cholera, leptospirosis, and erysipelas.

Lambs

LAMBS CAN BE hand-raised either by choice or by necessity. They are generally quite easy to raise, and it is enjoyable to do so. We do not know of any sheep rancher who has not, at one time or another, had to feed a lamb by hand—or farm it out to someone else to raise.

BUYING AND RAISING "EXTRA" LAMBS

Some sheepmen prefer their ewes to nurse only one lamb, so it will grow up quickly and extra fat. Ewes often have twins, so sometimes it is possible to contact sheep breeders ahead of lambing time, offering to buy these extra lambs soon after birth. In other instances, a ewe may have triplet lambs. There is a breed of sheep called Finn-sheep, known for having larger litters of lambs—often three or four, instead

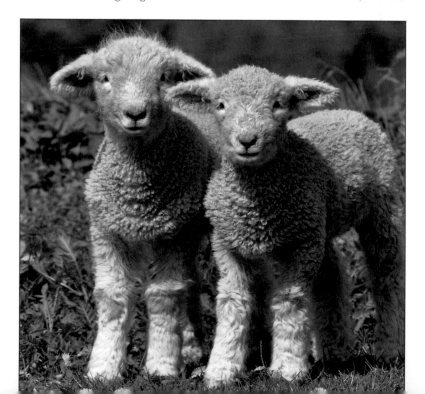

of the more normal single or twins. Ewes have only two teats so, of course, these extra lambs can also often be purchased shortly after birth. Buying these extra lambs can either be a quick start into the sheep business, or they might just furnish the family with a supply of lamb for the freezer.

Orphaned or rejected lambs are also readily available. However, the price should be quite a bit lower than for lambs that have had a good start on the ewe. The stress of an unloving start in life can make a lamb harder to raise successfully. Many sheepmen give these "bummers" or orphans away, just to save their time.

All lambs should receive the colostrum, or first milk, from their dam or a nurse ewe for three days, before they are taken home. This is very important because the colostrum not only contains a laxative to stimulate the bowel of the lamb, but it also has antibodies which help protect the newborn lamb from sickness. There is no substitute for natural colostrum. If ewe colostrum cannot be fed, use cow or goat colostrum, but be sure the lamb does receive colostrum, or its chances of living are reduced by about 70 percent.

The newborn lamb will usually drink about four ounces of milk every four hours. When possible, this milk should be goat milk, as it is much more digestible than either cow milk or powdered milk replacers. If a powdered milk replacer or cow milk must be fed, at least try to keep the lamb on goat milk for the first two weeks. After this time, it will be much stronger and more able to take on the harsher milk.

As the lamb increases in size and strength, increase its milk slowly. It is nothing short of amazing how fast lambs grow! At birth, they are the size of a smallish cat. In a week, they look like a little, rough, tough sheep, with a very active wagging tail.

No matter how tempting, do not keep the lamb in the house unless it has been chilled or is weak. These "house-pet" lambs very soon become a nuisance, dancing on the couch, upsetting tables and plants, and leaping on guests. Lambs are quite suited for barn life, as long as they are strong, dry, and in a well-bedded, draft-free pen.

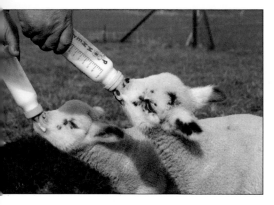

Lambs do quite well nursing on a lamb nipple fitted over the end of a 12-ounce pop bottle. A lamb nipple is much smaller than a calf nipple and made of a thinner rubber, making it easier for the smaller lambs to grasp and suck. It is a good idea to tuck a rubber band between the bottle and the nipple. This provides an airway, making it impossible for the hungry lamb to suck so hard that it creates a vacuum in the bottle, collapsing the nipple and making nursing impossible.

Be sure the lamb never gets quite its fill. Overfed lambs quickly come down with severe diarrhea which can kill them. The lamb's sides should be nice and round when feeding is done, but they should not pop out as though the lamb were bloated.

ENCOURAGING EWE TO TAKE REJECTED OR ADOPTED LAMB

If you have a flock of sheep, sooner or later, one of the ewes will reject a lamb, or perhaps a ewe will have more lambs than she can nurse, requiring the transfer of one lamb to a foster mother with a single lamb and plenty of milk.

Very few ewes will just accept such a transfer or begin taking care of a rejected lamb without much human help. But, with a bit of knowledge and some persistence, the ewe can be encouraged to do it.

Ewes know their own lambs primarily by smell, and they can tell one of their own lambs from the other in the same way. Therefore, it's necessary to make the lambs acceptable to the ewe by scent.

If she has only one lamb that she is nursing and taking care of, often you can place a second lamb with it in a small pen, away from the ewe for a few hours. Let their scents mingle and, perhaps, smear a little urine from the original lamb on the forehead and tail of the new lamb.

Then, with the ewe separated from the flock, give her a pail of feed and let the lambs come to nurse. You will have to watch her at first, as she may kick and butt both lambs a little in confusion. A couple of kicks or butts will discourage both lambs. But, usually, due to the distraction the feed provides, she will soon stop sniffing and begin eating, while the lambs nurse. If the kicking persists, smear some camphor on the ewe's nose, and also on the lambs. This will mask all smells for a while. You may have to restrain the ewe a few times if she is very kicky, but she usually begins to accept both lambs in a day or two.

Never leave lambs with a ewe that shows any sign of treating the lambs badly. It is much safer to place them in a separate pen between feedings for a while, until the ewe accepts them. An angry ewe often will kill lambs.

Another trick in switching lambs is to remove the skin from a stillborn lamb, placing it on the back of a foster lamb, then giving the ewe back "her" baby (by scent). This often works, but is quite messy for a few days. Be sure to tie the skin in place well, but not too tightly.

THE CHILLED LAMB

Due to the time of year the ewe flock lambs (December to March), lambs often become chilled soon after birth. It is best if "close-up" ewes (those close to delivery) are moved to a warm pen, even if it must be heated by a heat lamp or ultraviolet heater. Unfortunately, few people can or will do this, so the lambs are left in a cold climate at birth.

Dry, active lambs can take a lot of cold, but when they are wet from birth fluid, they are very vulnerable to chilling, especially if they are a bit weak or if the ewe doesn't get them cleaned off right away.

A chilled lamb cannot warm itself up nor dry itself off. It soon becomes motionless. The ewe often rejects its own lamb at this point. Without immediate help, the lamb will certainly die.

On discovering a chilled lamb, no matter how bad off it seems, quickly immerse it, all but the nose and mouth, in quite warm water. Keep the water warm, adding more hot water as needed, while a dry heat source is prepared. We have used a cardboard box, 18 by 18 inches with a heating pad in the bottom, an electric blanket (protect from shock and damage to the blanket by using a heavy towel around the damp lamb), the oven (keep the door open, temperature around 100°F, and constant supervision) and an incubator. As soon as the dry heat source is warm enough, remove the lamb from the water bath, and vigorously rub it dry. Really rub too! It will help restore circulation and also duplicate "mother love" to the lamb, encouraging it to move about.

Place the lamb in the warm place, turning it and rubbing it from time to time. If possible, steal a little of the ewe's colostrum, warm it to body temperature, and get it into the lamb.

TUBE-FEEDING

Many times, a chilled lamb will have lost the sucking reflex. Of course, the lamb cannot suck from a nipple, and forcing milk down the lamb's throat can kill it. So, when possible, the lamb should be tube-fed. This means that a small flexible tube is pushed down the lamb's throat, slowly and gently, and a syringe full of milk attached to the upper end of the tube is slowly discharged into the lamb's stomach. It is easy to learn to do this, and it is quite effective in livening up a chilled lamb. A lamb should be given about 30 cc of colostrum every two hours, until it is again lively and sucking. At this point, it can be returned to its mother. Be watchful for nonacceptance on her part, and also rechilling of the lamb. If at all possible, always provide artificial warmth for the ewe and lambs for a day or two.

If a lamb must be entirely hand-fed, here is a basic chart to follow. Please keep in mind, however, that some lambs will need more food and some less, depending on the individual. If a lamb seems to be gaining too slowly and feels thin, gradually increase the feed. If it seems too full or begins to have diarrhea, cut down on the amount fed.

The key to feeding lambs is to feed them enough to keep them gaining weight smoothly, and not so much as to cause diarrhea. Lambs will begin to nibble on hay at about a week of age, but they do not eat very much hay or grain until they are about three weeks old. However, both should be available to encourage eating solid food.

FEEDING SCHEDULE: BIRTH THROUGH WEANING

	Birth to 1 week	1 to 3 weeks	3 to 5 weeks	5 weeks to weaning
Milk	4 to 8 ounces	8 to 16 ounces	16 ounces	16 ounces
How often	every 2 to 3 hours	3 times daily	3 times daily	2 times daily
Hay	...	free choice	free choice	free choice
Grain (mixed)	...	free choice	free choice	free choice

SYMPTOMS OF TROUBLE— AND WHAT TO DO

DIARRHEA

This is the most common problem with hand-raised lambs. Too often, well-meaning owners give the lamb all it wants to eat. They feel that this way, the lamb will do better and grow faster. Even the lamb's own mother does not let it eat all it wants. Instead, the wise ewe simply walks off, leaving the lamb sniffing around with drops of milk on its nose.

At each feeding, you should check under the lamb's tail. At birth, the lamb has a slightly pasty, blackish stool which soon turns yellowish. It is a day or so before the manure takes on the "berry" look. Once this has happened, the manure should never again look pasty or loose.

If it does, try cutting down the amount of milk given at each feeding for a day, and see if the stool returns to normal. This usually works. After the passage of several solid stools, the milk can be increased slowly to almost the amount that caused the diarrhea.

If the stool does not tighten up, give the lamb two to four ounces of kaolin-pectin (depending on the size of the lamb), every two hours until a normal stool is passed. Do not cheat, thinking that one or two doses will be enough. If the diarrhea is allowed to go on, the intestinal tract becomes highly irritated, allowing the growth of damaging bacteria. The intestinal tract becomes infected, and the diarrhea will continue and worsen until it is nearly impossible to save the lamb.

If the kaolin-pectin does not stop the diarrhea within 12 hours, consult with your veterinarian. He may prescribe antibiotics, or put the lamb on an electrolyte solution. An electrolyte solution is made up of salts and chemicals, normal to the body, that are lost when dehydration takes place. If these electrolytes are not replaced and the animal is dehydrated, it will often die.

Electrolyte solutions can be given orally in the place of milk for a day, or given intravenously or intraperitoneally (in the abdominal cavity) if the lamb is severely dehydrated.

The lamb with diarrhea should be kept clean and warm, even if it must be brought into the house in a box. Fly strike, an infestation of fly larvae, is common in lambs, if they are born in warmer weather, so flies must be kept away from the fouled wool with a fly repellent.

PNEUMONIA

Other than starvation, pneumonia has been called the number one killer of baby lambs. Pneumonia is a sneaky killer. It is commonly thought that poorly kept animals are most susceptible. One immediately thinks of those lambs kept in a cold, dreary barn. But, unfortunately, well-cared-for animals are just about as likely to get pneumonia as those in cold barns. Animals in the early stages of pneumonia seldom cough—another fooler. Any lamb that suddenly acts listless or a little "slow" should immediately have its temperature taken. If it is above 102°F, antibiotics should be started immediately. Tomorrow might be too late, as pneumonia can kill very quickly.

If one lamb in a flock has pneumonia, isolate it and carefully watch the others for the slightest abnormal action. If such action is noticed, take the temperature. Sometimes pneumonia in lambs is so fast-acting that an apparently healthy lamb (though running a temperature) can be dead within 12 hours. If more than one lamb comes down with pneumonia, call your veterinarian at once.

Antibiotic therapy will save a good number of lambs with pneumonia. But *never* just give one or two injections, even if the lamb suddenly becomes well. There will be some organisms left in the body that have not yet been killed and, without continued injections, they may well overcome the body again. This time they will be very hard to destroy.

FREEZING AND FROSTBITE

Any lamb that has been born in freezing weather and has been brought in to hand-raise, especially because of rejection or the death of its mother, should be checked very carefully for signs of freezing or frostbite. Generally, lambs are quite resistant to these conditions, due to their nice coat of wool. But damp wool can quickly freeze, causing problems.

Especially check the ears, legs, and tail. If any swelling or stiffness is noticed, immediately immerse the affected part in lukewarm water, and keep it there for half-an-hour. After that time, massage the lamb thoroughly with a warm towel and place it in a warm, dry box. Keep a careful watch to make sure there is not a lot of swelling of that part which was frozen. If swelling does occur, contact your veterinarian. He can give cortisone injections and give you more tips on daily care and treatment to fit the situation.

If nothing is done for a lamb that has been frozen or severely frostbitten, the part will swell, turn dark, become gangrenous and drop off. This includes ears, feet, legs, and tail.

GENERAL CARE

After the first week on a bottle, lambs are quite easy to raise. If there are several lambs being raised, they can be placed together in one pen. Sheep are flock animals and they are much happier if they have company. Be sure there is adequate room, however, so that the pen stays clean and dry and that there is no fighting over hay and grain as the lambs grow older.

Feed hay out of low mangers with slanted slots for the heads to go through, or else they will drag out a lot of hay and waste it. Grain can be fed out of long, low troughs, about 12 or 18 inches high. The trough should not be just set on the ground, or the lambs will walk in it and manure in it, increasing the chances of their picking up internal parasites.

At the age of 8 to 10 weeks, the lambs should receive a vaccination to protect them against enterotoxemia, or overeating disease. This disease most often strikes very well-fed lambs, and is nearly always fatal once symptoms show.

Sometime between three weeks and eight weeks, the lambs should have their tails docked. This is essential, not for appearance, but for the lambs' own well-being. Long-tailed sheep often have fecal material trapped between body and tail. This becomes damp and foul, attracting flies. The flies lay eggs, which soon hatch out into maggots. These larvae soon attack not only the foul manure, but the sheep's body as well. In a week's time, they can actually devour an adult sheep, from the inside out. Unfortunately, there are few signs of trouble until the sheep is very far gone.

Docking is a very simple matter of an emasculator (the instrument used when castrating horses) is applied to the tail. This not only quickly cuts the tail off, but crushes the blood vessels at the same time, preventing loss of blood. This instrument is expensive, so it is usually best to take the lamb to your veterinarian or to an experienced sheepman in the area. Using a hatchet or chisel to dock the tail is dangerous.

Kids

DAIRY GOATS ARE among the most useful of all the creatures, providing meat, milk, and companionship. They are also very
easy to hand-raise. This is how many people get started in goats—that
irresistible kid, followed by another, and another, and many more. In
fact, few goat raisers let the kids nurse on their mother. The milk can
usually be sold for a good price, so the kids are usually bottle or pan-
fed, and weaning is done at an early age. All kids, no matter how they
are raised, should have the colostrum or mother's first milk for three
days. This milk not only provides a laxative, moving "stale" manure
through the kid's digestive tract, but gives it antibodies to help fight off
serious illnesses early in life.

It is also very important to be sure that the kid's navel has been
dipped in iodine very soon after birth, as goats are very susceptible
to infection in the joints, caused by organisms gaining access to the
body through the umbilical cord. Sometimes these organisms are
semidormant for months, until they flare up into a severe infection,
often crippling the goat.

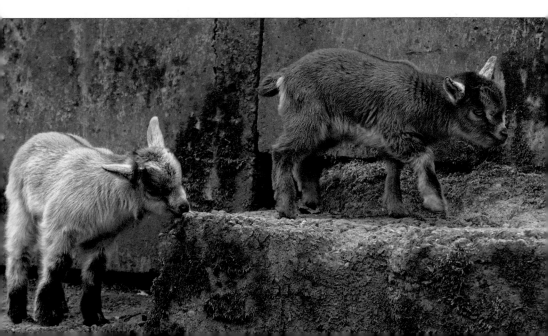

CARE AND FEEDING OF THE NEWBORN KID

Most kids are quite small at birth, weighing between 5 and 10 pounds. Single births, most often occurring in first fresheners (does giving birth for the first time) usually weigh more than do multiple births. At birth kids are a little delicate, but soon gain strength after a little care, preferably from the mother.

Many goat breeders never let the kids nurse on the doe at all, removing the kids before they have even been dried off. We do not do this on our farm. All normal kids are kept in a separate stall with their mother for four days. We feel that this gives the kids a much better start in life. One important factor is that the kids snack from the doe many, many times daily, instead of having to settle for the two or three feedings the owner can manage to provide. Very frequently, small feedings are better digested and more fully utilized.

After four days, if desired, the kids can be removed to a kid stall that is dry and draft-free, containing four or five kids of equal size. Here they can be bottle-fed, if necessary.

Once more, we do things a bit differently than the "norm." Instead of feeding milk replacer, which is very hard to digest and causes digestive upsets, we place all kids that are going to be kept, either for sale or for herd replacements, on nurse does. A nurse doe can be any doe that is hard to hand-milk, is not a good milker, or has had a mastitis problem. We have not, so far, had a mastitis flare-up in a nurse doe that has had a previous history of mastitis during a hand-milked lactation. Do not, however, place kids on a doe with an active case of mastitis, as it could harm them.

TRAINING THE NURSE DOE

There are three very important things to watch while training a doe to be a foster mother:

— Do not let her kick the kids.
— Do not let her loose with the kids unsupervised, until she is "mothering" them.
— Do not let nursing kids run with the milking herd.

It is natural for a doe to reject any kids that are not her own. When a hungry kid is persistent, a doe can get vicious, biting, butting, and kicking the kid. Tie the doe snugly, and give her a good big pan of grain to chew on. Be handy, both to supervise the kid and to keep her from kicking it.

Repeat this three times daily, until the doe makes no move to kick at the kid. When she begins to accept it, she will squat, spreading her legs, making it easy for the kid to nurse.

When she reaches this point, you can try letting her have a little more room to move about. Either tie her a bit longer, or do not put her head in the stanchion. When she makes no move to kick or butt the kid, you can try just turning her loose in a small pen with the kid at feeding time, while both of them eat. If she does not try to harm the kid after a day's time, you can be quite sure she has adopted it.

You should, however, check the doe's bag daily for a week, to be sure that the kid is nursing. (If it is, at least one side will be quite flabby.)

If the doe is any kind of milker, she should be able to handle at least two kids, and quite probably three or more. Ideally, she should remain nearly "sucked dry," but not be completely dry. However, if only one kid is nursing, it will not be able to drink all the milk the

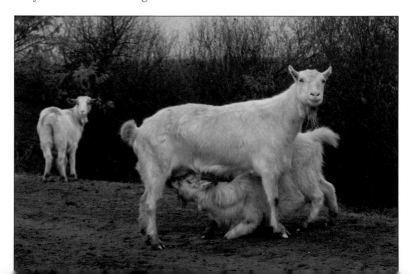

doe produces, and you will have to milk her dry twice daily, or she will be in danger of getting mastitis (inflammation of the udder). If more than one kid is to be nursed by the nurse doe, it is easiest to introduce all of them at once, instead of one at a time.

THE BOTTLE-FED KID

Sometimes it is not possible to find, or use, a nurse doe. The next best solution, in my opinion, is bottle-feeding the kid. When drinking from the bottle, the kid holds its head in a natural upright position and sucks small amounts of milk. When drinking from a pail or pan, the kid has a tendency to gulp large amounts of milk with its head held down. This may cause the milk to end up in the wrong stomach (goats have four), which can cause bloating and severe indigestion.

At birth, the normal kid weighs between 5 and 10 pounds and is quite active for short periods of time. Soon after birth, it is vital to be sure the kid receives at least two ounces of the doe's first milk, colostrum. The kid will usually drink soon after birth, and will be hungry every three hours thereafter. If the kid seems a little weak or backward, feed it small amounts every two or three hours. If the kid is larger, and more vigorous, the amount fed can be increased to six ounces or so, and three feedings a day will be enough.

As the kid grows during the first week, the milk should be increased. Most kids can drink eight ounces or more three times daily by the time they are a week old. The kid should never be fed so much that it is completely full. It should always be a little hungry when it finishes eating. The stomach should look full, but not stuffed.

The best bottle to use for the kid is a 12-ounce pop bottle fitted with a lamb nipple. The lamb nipple is a black rubber nipple, smaller than a calf nipple, and longer than a human baby bottle nipple. The lamb nipple is tough and slips snugly over the end of most pop bottles. As the kid nurses, the nipple has a tendency to collapse as a vacuum forms in the bottle. This is easily remedied by placing a loop of

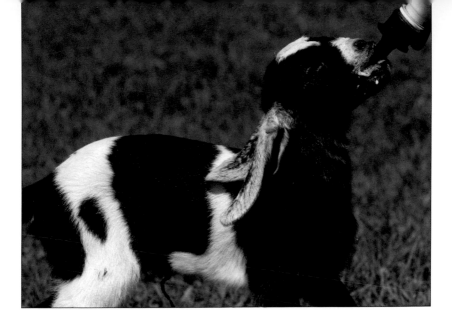

a small rubber band between the nipple and the bottle. This lets air into the bottle as the kid sucks, preventing the nipple from collapsing, and allowing easier nursing.

THE WEAK OR CHILLED KID

Some kids are born quite weak, or are severely chilled soon after birth, leaving them stiff and cold. These kids very seldom have any sucking reflex left and will certainly die without help. As soon as such a kid is discovered, it is vital to bring it into the house at once. Soak it in warm water and massage the whole kid until it appears more active. At this point, dry the kid well, and place it in a very warm box.

Then warm some colostrum, and prepare to tube-feed the kid. Necessary equipment includes a small diameter, flexible plastic or rubber tube several inches long, and a syringe 12 cc or larger. The largest diameter tube used on newborn kids should be the size of a pencil. Larger tubes will choke the kid or make it fight the feeding.

Anyone who has a doe expecting kids would be wise to buy a French catheter (feeding tube) from a veterinarian. The cost is usually under a dollar, and that tube is worth much, much more when that special kid is born weak, at an inconvenient time, such as 1:00 AM on a Sunday morning—and the veterinarian is not available.

The tube should be gently but firmly slipped down the kid's throat, as its head is tipped slightly upward. The kid should begin swallowing as the tube is slipped down its throat. If it should begin coughing, immediately withdraw the tube and try again, as it is possible that the feeding tube might be going down the kid's trachea, into the lung. If milk were to be directed into the lungs, it would probably kill the kid, so caution is necessary in tube-feeding.

As soon as the tube is down the throat (judge by the length of the tube compared to the length of the kid's neck), attach the syringe full of milk (warmed to the kid's body temperature—approximately 102°F), and slowly inject the milk into the feeding tube. This should be repeated several times, until about 30 to 40 cc of milk have been fed. Then, slowly withdraw the tube. Generally this small amount of colostrum, coupled with the warming up, will soon perk the kid up enough so that it regains the sucking instinct. Then it can be fed more via the bottle within an hour's time. As soon as the kid acts hungry, offer the nipple, and keep doing this until the kid sucks. The milk must be warm, and the kid must not be forced.

Sometimes it is necessary to give the kid two or more tube-feedings before the sucking reflex returns. Just keep the kid warm, and tube-feed every two hours, and chances are good that the kid will soon come around.

FEEDING SCHEDULE: BIRTH THROUGH WEANING

	Birth to 1 week	1 to 3 weeks	3 to 5 weeks	5 weeks to weaning
Milk	4 to 8 ounces	8 to 16 ounces	16 ounces	16 ounces
How often	every 4 hours	3 times daily	2 times daily	2 times daily
Hay	...	free choice	free choice	free choice
Grain	...	free choice	free choice	free choice
Calf Manna		free choice	free choice	1 cup daily

When the kid is fed entirely by hand, you can follow the chart. Keep in mind, though, that each kid is an individual, and that some kids will need more—or less—depending on the individual. If a kid seems to gain weight too slowly, and feels thin between feedings, gradually increase the feed. If it seems too full, or begins to have diarrhea, cut down on the amount fed at each feeding.

SYMPTOMS OF TROUBLE— AND WHAT TO DO

CONSTIPATION

One of the first problems to watch out for in newborn kids is constipation. Often these kids have not nursed well soon after birth, so they have not had the laxative in the colostrum which pushes the "stale" manure through the intestines. This manure is very tarry and sticky and tends to constipate. It is very important to note the passage of this bowel movement, which will be quite dark and sticky. If this is not passed, it is wise to give the kid a mild enema.

If a kid suddenly appears weak soon after birth and was previously active and hungry, constipation should be suspected. Search for any dark stools in the pen, or clinging to the kid's tail. If none are found, or only small amounts, give the kid an enema at once. If the kid is left untreated until a later time, it might die due to the absorption of toxic material from the bowel.

Also, the constipated kid usually has an abdomen that appears "full." It will feel slightly "squishy soft."

An enema usually brings about a bowel movement quickly and relieves the kid.

DIARRHEA

Diarrhea is quite common in kids that get too much milk. If that situation is immediately corrected, the kid will probably pass one or two loose bowel movements, and then quickly return to normal. But, too often, the kid is fed more milk before the condition is noticed, and the diarrhea worsens. And, too often, the kid is given an injection of antibiotics or a pill for what ails it and still fed the regular amount of milk. By this time, the kid's bowels are severely irritated, and the diarrhea becomes very hard to treat.

So it is obvious that diarrhea should be watched for at each feeding and, if it is noted, the next feeding should be cut in half, and warm water substituted for the other half of the milk.

By the time the next feeding is due, the diarrhea should have stopped. If the kid is in a lightly bedded pen or box, changes in the manure are easily noted.

If the diarrhea has not stopped when it's time for the next feedings, give the kid two to four ounces of kaolin-pectin then, and every two hours thereafter, until the diarrhea subsides. If it does not slow down or stop after four hours and three doses of kaolin-pectin, replace all milk being fed with an oral electrolyte solution. As the diarrhea continues, the kid not only loses body fluids (regardless of the milk fed), but also body salts and chemicals. Not only must the fluid be replaced, but those natural body chemicals as well, for without them the kid will continue to have severe diarrhea until it weakens and dies.

A kid that has been on oral electrolytes and kaolin-pectin for 24 hours and still has not improved should be examined by a veterinarian. Sometimes treatment with antibiotics or intestinal sulfas, or intravenous electrolyte therapy is necessary to save the kid's life.

On occasion, kids will have diarrhea when they are older. Quite often this is caused by an internal parasite, *coccidia*. Coccidiosis is commonly present in older goats, but they have become more or less immune to it. However, kids are severely affected by it, often dying if treatment is not given.

Diarrhea in older kids can be caused by overfeeding. If this is not the case, take a sample of the loose stool to a veterinarian to examine for the presence of *coccidia*. Treatment with intestinal sulfas or Corid is common, and quite effective. If the kid is found to have coccidiosis, treatment at monthly intervals should be given, as *coccidia* are quite hardy. Follow the advice of your veterinarian.

PNEUMONIA

Many kids die from pneumonia each year. Kids with pneumonia generally lose their appetites quickly—perhaps eating well in the morning, but not appearing hungry at night. Do not look for coughing; few kids with pneumonia cough—they don't live long enough to cough. And don't wait for a kid that "just isn't hungry" in the afternoon to "get better" by evening or morning. *Take the temperature at once!* If it is over 102°F, suspect pneumonia, and begin treatment with pen-strep or another broad-spectrum antibiotic. If the kid is responding, it usually acts much better within 24 hours, and its temperature is usually normal or at least much lower than it was. Continue the antibiotics, even if the kid acts perfectly normal. If this is not done, the kid will probably relapse with the pneumonia, and possibly not respond to the antibiotic again, as the pneumonia organisms will have gained resistance to it.

If the kid does not show marked improvement within 12 hours, contact your veterinarian.

PARASITES

Goats are prone to intestinal parasites, namely worms and *coccidia*. Every goat should be checked by a veterinarian at least once a year. If necessary, a worming program can be started, following the examination. Do not think that you will see worms in the manure if the goat is wormy, or that a fat goat cannot have worms. Both are false ideas.

Goats do get lice during the winter months, so once a month it is good to dust all goats in the barn with a louse powder containing rotenone, a quite harmless natural insecticide. And, as they can get worms, well-cared-for goats *do* get lice, and can be run down by their numbers before any signs of baldness or scratching are noticed. So take care, and prevent trouble by preventative dusting.

VACCINATIONS

Kids should be vaccinated against tetanus at three weeks of age. This disease is quite common in goats and is usually fatal. They should also be vaccinated against enterotoxemia (overeating disease) at a young age—five to seven weeks. This disease is very common in well-fed goats, which most hand-raised goats are. It is also usually fatal.

In some areas white muscle disease is common. If it is seen in your area (your veterinarian can tell you this), vaccinate kids soon after birth.

It is wise to ask your veterinarian if there are any other diseases in your particular area he would recommend vaccinating against, as some diseases are common only to certain parts of the country. You don't want to vaccinate that poor kid against everything possible—it would look like a pincushion with legs!

GENERAL CARE

Goat kids are very hardy once they are a week old, and need only basic care. A draft-free shelter, be it a barn or large dog house, regular feedings, fresh water, a salt block, and reasonable supervision are all they require. At the age of three to four days, most kids begin growing

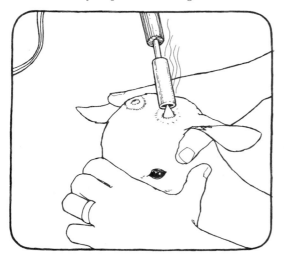

horns. These tiny horn buds can be felt on the top of the head, hidden by hair. Some people think that goats are pretty with horns, or more "natural," but horns on goats are very dangerous—not so much for people as for other goats, and even dangerous to the wearer itself. Horns catch on things, even a goat's own collar, causing many broken necks, strangulations, and deaths. Those horns can also accidentally put out a child's eye or tear an adult's cheek. To be safe, the kid should be disbudded as soon as the tiny, sharp horn buds can be felt.

Disbudding is easiest done by the use of a red-hot dehorning iron at 3–4 days or earlier. Every goat breeder should have a dehorning iron. If you do not, call the nearest goat breeder and ask him or her to disbud your kid.

The red-hot iron is applied to first one horn bud, then the other, leaving a copper-colored indented ring around each one. The kid will scream and yell during the procedure, but then will quickly forget that anything happened, and be as trusting and friendly as ever. Remember that you may be saving its life by having it disbudded.

If the kid is a buck and will not be used for breeding purposes, it can be castrated at the same time it is disbudded. Remember that only the bucks with the best bloodlines should be used for breeding. Don't keep a buck entire just because he is "cute" or "a pretty color." Castration is safest done by the use of an emasculatome, a "Burdizzo" (a clamp that crushes the cords and blood vessels to the testicles, causing them to shrink up), or by surgery.

Goats are very fastidious and will not eat soiled feed or drink dirty water. One "nanny berry" in the drinking water will keep most goats from drinking until they are dehydrated. The solution to this is the keyhole manger (see illustration). Both water and feed are reached through the keyhole, eliminating contamination and preventing the waste of feed.

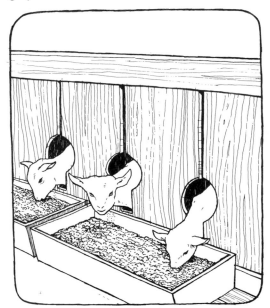

Crias

BABY CAMELIDS; LLAMAS, ALPACAS, and VICUNAS

LLAMAS, ALPACAS, AND vicunas are becoming more and more popular in this country, raised primarily for their luxuriant, thick coats. The wool is spun and made into yarn of the finest and softest kind. These animals, primarily llamas, are also raised for guard animals for flocks of sheep. They are hardy, beautiful, and easy to raise, making them very popular with hobby farmers.

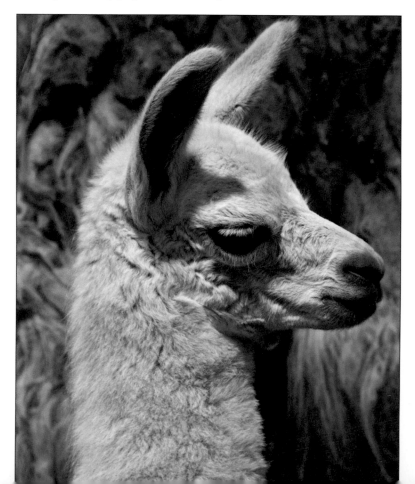

CARE AND FEEDING OF NEWBORN CRIAS

Most births occur during the daytime, which gives the owner a much better chance of being on hand for the birth. Single births are the norm, with twins being quite rare. It's best to keep the pregnant female in a grassy, clean pasture in good weather, prior to birth or if the weather is unstable, a large, warm, well bedded box stall is the best alternative. Most females give birth and take care of the cria unaided. Most strong crias get up to their feet and nurse within three hours or less of birth.

Be sure to dip the umbilical stump in iodine or Betadine immediately after birth and then again in a few hours to avoid infection. An umbilical infection can be very serious and kill a newborn cria, as well as leading to later, very serious problems.

Make sure the cria is dried off immediately after birth, especially the head and nose cleaned of any fluids or clinging afterbirth. If the cria seems struggling for breath, hold it up by its hind legs to let the fluid drain, then vigorously rub its sides with a dry towel.

Most females readily mother their crias, but on occasion, one will have a very sensitive udder or simply NOT want to be a mother. Without nursing, the cria will soon weaken and die.

THE HAND RAISED CRIA

The first milk for a cria should be its mother's colostrum or first milk. Sometimes you can convince the female to let you milk her by tying her in a corner and having a helper hold her against the stall wall while you milk into a bottle. If not, you should have on hand before any births are due some frozen goat colostrum. Warm the frozen colostrum and pour about 4 ounces into a bottle with a lamb nipple on it or a human baby bottle. Most crias will soon learn to nurse from the bottle. If the cria is weak and/or unwilling to nurse, tube feeding with a French catheter and 60 cc syringe. Hold the tube next to the cria and measure from the corner of its mouth to about the middle back of its ribs. Then draw a mark on the tube with a permanent marker. Cut the catheter to fit on the syringe. Lubricate the tube with milk (the cria will be more prone to suck than if you use KY Jelly). Slowly insert the tube into the cria's mouth, letting it swallow as you gently but firmly push the tube down its throat. It is very rare that the tube will get into the lungs, but if the cria begins to cough, immediately withdraw the tube and begin again. When the tube is in place in the stomach, use the syringe to slowly deposit the warmed milk. A normal sized cria will take from between 4-6 oz of milk every four hours for the first two days, with the amount increasing thereafter. Thankfully, usually once the cria is stronger and a little older, it will usually readily accept a bottle.

If the cria is chilled it can not warm itself despite the woolly coat. Weak and chilled crias should be warmed by a soak (with the head held above the water) in a warm bathtub or a heat lamp carefully monitored to avoid too much heat. A chilled or weak cria usually needs to be tube fed for a time or two until it recovers. If this is the only problem, it can often be returned to nurse on its mother upon complete recovery. Do monitor the female, as sometimes the mother rejects the baby and can even harm it.

A cria should be bottle fed about 4-6 ounces of milk for the first few days, feeding at least three times a day; four is best, with hours divided evenly. After that, you can gradually increase the feedings by 2 ounces and reduce the frequency of feedings to two or three feedings a day, depending on the cria. Goat milk is best, after mother's milk. If this is impossible, there are some good powdered camelid (camel family; llama, alpaca, vicuna) milk replacers available. Be sure the powder is extremely well mixed with the warm water prior to feeding to avoid intestinal upset leading to diarrhea.

Usually once the cria is warm and has been fed twice, it is quite strong and getting hungry in between feedings and will be fine with good care.

Monitor the stools of the cria, making first sure that there *are* stools. Constipation is occasionally seen in newborn crias and untreated, this can kill them. If the cria suddenly appears weak and no bowel movements have been seen, give the cria an enema at once, using a warmed Fleet enema. This usually brings about a quick bowel movement and relief for the cria.

Diarrhea is quite common in crias that get too much milk. If that is the case, immediately reduce the amount of milk fed. By the time the next feeding is due, the diarrhea should have stopped. If not, give the cria four ounces of kaolin-pectin then and substitute the milk feeding with a feeding of liquid electrolytes (available at your veterinarian's office). This should bring about quick relief from simple milk-overload. If not, call your veterinarian, as diarrhea can quickly weaken and kill a cria.

Pups

ONE OF THE most familiar domestic animals whose baby or babies are often in need of human raising is the dog. The chief reason for this is that there are so many dogs—and dog lovers—in this country. The odds dictate that out of the thousands of litters of puppies born in the United States each year, many pups will need human help to survive. Of course, many people just let those pups die—or kill them. But a lot of people take over the responsibility of raising the puppies themselves. And it really is a responsibility!

THE ORPHANED, REJECTED, OR "NEEDY" PUP

When pups must be hand-raised, it is usually because their mother has died or cannot raise them for some reason. Some bitches (the correct name for female dogs) get mastitis, or an infection in their breasts, a

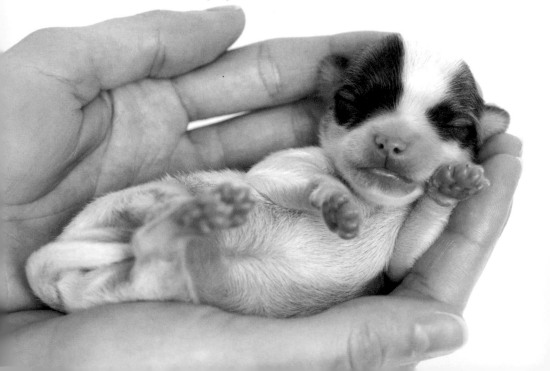

uterine infection, or have no milk for the puppies. Other bitches just have too many pups to take care of. Whatever the reason, you might suddenly find yourself the foster parent of from 1 to 13 puppies!

Raising these puppies is a lot of work, but it can be very rewarding. Be prepared to feed them every two hours, day and night for two weeks. There can be no cheating. One feeding missed, and puppies are likely to die.

Not only must the puppies be fed, but they must be stimulated with a warm, damp washcloth to make them urinate and defecate. This has to be done or they will not eliminate as needed, and soon will become constipated and toxic. Keep the puppies in a warm box, heated, if necessary, to keep them comfortable.

Very young puppies are easiest fed by the stomach tube. This feeding method may not seem as "mothering" as feeding with a bottle, but is much faster, and when you have 10 hungry puppies to feed at three in the morning, I'll bet you'll choose "fast" over "mothering" in about one day's time!

Tube-feeding is quite easy to learn, and quite safe, provided that you do take your time at first and pay attention to what you are doing.

First of all, you must determine how much milk each pup should get. The following chart can give a rough idea, but do keep in mind that all pups are different and these figures are just a starting point. Puppies should look full, but not stuffed after each feeding. Their abdomens should look rounded, but not like someone stuffed a tennis ball in there! Puppies should gain weight steadily. The hip bones and backbone should not jut out, nor should all boney framework be covered by gross amounts of "puppy fat." Judge feeding amounts by what the individual pup is doing on what it is fed. If it does not gain weight and does not look full, gradually increase the amount given each time. If it gets loose bowels, decrease the milk.

Obtain several disposable syringes of the correct size (at least large enough to hold one pup's feeding from birth to one week—remember that the birth amount will increase by about one-third in a week's time), and a feeding tube. A French catheter or the right size

for the breed can be most successfully used. You can get these supplies very easily from your veterinarian.

We prefer to use goat milk for raising puppies, as it is highly
digestible and no mixing is necessary. There are powdered puppy
formulas on the market that can be used if goat milk is not available.
Milk fed the first two weeks should be warmed to body temperature,
and care should be taken to keep the milk that is fed to the last pup
as warm as—no warmer nor cooler—the milk that was fed to the first
pup. Puppies are prone to chilling, and giving cold milk can easily
bring on a chill.

A good way to keep the milk warm is to set a small jar of milk, just
enough for one feeding, in a pan of warm water. The larger amount
of warm water will keep the milk at an even temperature during the
feeding, without the need to rewarm it.

When tube-feeding for the first few times, it is best to insert the
tube *before* filling it; if it is inserted down the trachea (leading to the
lungs), droplets of milk may leak into the lungs and kill the pup. Usually, the tube slips right down the pup's throat into the stomach, but
an inexperienced person could miss. Don't shove it, and don't expect
the pup to do all the work. If you get the pup to swallow the tube, there
is no chance of incorrect placement.

When the tube is well down the throat (judge by matching the
length of tube with the length of the pup's neck), slowly deposit the
milk. Do not push the syringe plunger in fast, as this will cause the
milk to spray in the stomach at a powerful rate, causing discomfort
and possibly indigestion. After all the milk has been given, slowly
withdraw the tube. No need to take all day over this, but don't just
yank it out either.

As you gain experience, it is best to fill the tube and attach it to the
syringe before inserting the stomach tube. This will prevent depositing air into the stomach, along with the milk. The air could cause
indigestion. Never begin depositing the milk until you are sure the
tube is down far enough. Too quick a trigger finger may cause drops of
milk to be inhaled by the pup, killing it.

AMOUNT TO FEED NEWBORN PUPS (BY SIZE)

Toy breeds (Chihuahua, Toy Poodle)	4 to 6 cc
Small breeds (Pug, Fox Terrier)	6 to 8 cc
Medium breeds (Cocker, Min. Poodle)	8 to 10 cc
Large breeds (Afghan, Collie)	10 to 12 cc
Very large breeds (St. Bernard, Newfoundland)	20 to 25 cc

Remember, as the pups grow, day by day, you must gradually increase their milk allotment, always keeping that tummy nice and round (but not bulging).

After each pup is fed, be sure to massage the genitals with a warm, damp, soft cloth, stimulating the mother's tongue. This is important, not only for cleanliness of the box, but for the health of the pups.

From the time you take on the raising of the puppies, you must keep them warm. This means keeping them in a box, lined with a cookie sheet, with a heating pad under the whole works, or a box with a heat lamp, or an incubator. They must have dependable, steady warmth to live.

It is easiest if the puppies are kept in the bedroom, which makes night feedings more convenient.

Be sure to keep a clean towel in the box to absorb any "accidents" and that will keep the puppies from becoming soiled.

Puppies may be fed with a bottle. Try to match the size of the bitch's nipples with that of the bottle's nipple. Tiny toy pups do best on a doll bottle with a *rubber* nipple (some doll bottles have plastic nipples and are not acceptable). Medium breed pups do well on a "Pet Nip" type nurser. Large and giant breed pups often do best on a human baby bottle.

Remember, *don't let the pups nurse until completely full.* Let them get comfortably full, but take the bottle away when you think they would drink a little more if you let them.

After they are two weeks old, begin adding some high-protein baby cereal to the milk, keeping it thin enough to go through the nipple.

As soon as their eyes open, the pups can be encouraged to take a little ground liver or mashed, hard-boiled egg yolk from your fingertip.

When the pups are three weeks of age, take a sample of their droppings to your veterinarian. Because they were stressed, hand-raised pups often have a heavy parasite load at this young age and must be wormed with a mild wormer. Do this only with your veterinarian's assistance, as many wormers are very toxic and might kill the pups instead of curing them.

SYMPTOMS OF TROUBLE— AND WHAT TO DO

DIARRHEA

Diarrhea is one of the greatest killers of young puppies. In many cases, young puppies that are "abandoned by their mothers" or "rejected," simply become dehydrated from diarrhea and crawl off to one corner of the nest in shock.

Diarrhea is seldom diagnosed in young nursing puppies because at this age, the bitch keeps all stools carefully cleaned up, often before they entirely leave the pup. Thus no one sees the loose stool, or guesses that the problem exists.

The initial diarrhea may have been caused by several things—too much milk, a uterine infection that changes the milk, or antibiotic residues in the bitch's milk from "preventative" antibiotic injections.

It is, of course, important to determine the cause of the diarrhea, but the most important thing is to recognize the fact that the pup or pups *do* have diarrhea.

Any pup that crawls away from the nest and seems cold should come under strong suspicion. This pup will usually cry, even when returned to the bitch. The pup will feel bony, and its skin will feel off—as if the pup has too much skin for its size. The area under its tail may appear yellowish, but not usually dirty (due to the bitch's clean-

FEEDING SCHEDULE: BIRTH THROUGH WEANING

	Birth to 1 week	1 to 2 weeks	2 to 3 weeks	3 to 5 weeks	5 to 8 weeks	8 weeks on
Milk	x	x	x	x	x	...
Hi-protein baby cereal	...	...	x	x	...	...
Ground liver	...	...	x	x	...	...
Puppy formula dry dog food	...	...	...	x	x	x
Feedings per day	12	12	8	6	3	3

ing tongue). The temperature will often be subnormal by the time anything wrong is noticed, as the pup often suffers for a day or longer before any trouble is suspected.

Often, such a pup can be saved if it is removed from the nest at once, and treatment is begun.

The hand-raised pup can also suffer from diarrhea, but its diarrhea is most often caused by indigestion—too much milk, a change in formula, or the like. Sometimes just reducing the amount of milk fed during the next meal is enough to straighten out the trouble. But, often additional treatment becomes necessary. If the pup continues drinking milk and is not treated at once for the diarrhea, it will soon end up like the pup described above—in shock, with a subnormal temperature, and close to death.

If started in time, treatment is often successful. As soon as you notice a pup acting strangely (not "running" in its sleep, jerking, or not appearing very hungry at meal time), immediately think of diarrhea and check for it. You can do this by massaging the rectal area with a warm damp cloth, encouraging the pup to defecate. Should a yellowish, watery, bubbly diarrhea appear instead of a pasty, formed stool, start treatment at once!

Give the pup half as much kaolin-pectin (with neomycin if possible) as its usual milk feeding. For instance, if you are giving 6 cc of milk, give it 3 cc of kaolin-pectin. Then, an hour later, give it as much oral electrolyte solution as you regularly do milk.

As the pup's diarrhea continues, not only does it lose precious body fluids, but also body salts and other chemicals. The electrolytes give the pup back all three, without further irritating the intestinal tract as milk would.

Give no milk until after the stool returns to normal, or for 24 hours. Continue giving the kaolin-pectin every 2 hours until relief is noticed, giving the electrolyte solution every other hour.

If no relief is noticed after eight hours, contact the veterinarian. The pup may need parenteral electrolytes (injectable) or additional antibiotic or sulfa treatment.

CONSTIPATION

Constipation is not as bad a problem in pups as it is in some other animals, but it is a good idea to be aware of it. If a puppy begins to act listless but appears full, with its abdomen rounded, give an enema at once, using as much warm soapy water as half its milk feeding. Therefore, if you are feeding 8 cc of milk, give the pup an enema with 4 cc of warm soapy water. An enema may be given with a number of things, but a baby ear syringe works well on many breeds. Use anything with a smooth tip that is about as thick as the pup's normal stool. Measure the amount of enema solution carefully, to be sure too much is not accidentally given.

Generally, one enema brings prompt relief and soon the pup is acting livelier and is hungry.

DISTEMPER

It is a good idea to give hand-raised pups an injection of gamma globulin at three weeks of age to protect them from distemper. Distemper is a disease of dogs affecting the central nervous system. Young pups are often seen with it. Early symptoms include mattered eyes, a crusty, mucous-encrusted nose and, often, diarrhea. Later on, the pup may lose the use of its tail, begin twitching a limb, have convulsions, refuse to eat, weaken, and stagger.

It is highly contagious. You can pick it up on your clothes or shoes on the street and bring it home to your new pups. And, with lessened immunity that results from drinking only a limited amount of their mother's milk, they can easily contract the disease. It is usually fatal, even with treatment.

GENERAL CARE

After the puppies are about three weeks old, they will require a larger box. A big refrigerator box is ideal. Their bed can be at one end of it, with their "potty" papers at the far end, away from their bed. Not only will this keep the blankets in their bed cleaner, but it will be the start of house-training them. Puppies do not like to be near their mess, so will do it as far from their bed as possible. We have had two-week-old puppies crawl out of the nest to "do their business" elsewhere before they could even see!

Between three weeks and weaning, the puppies will suddenly become a bunch of mess-makers. It doesn't seem possible that they could dirty up their box in so short a time, but can they! To fight this and keep them smelling nice, shred up newspapers in narrow strips. This will cling to the stools and absorb wetness.

When they are eight weeks old, they can move outside (sooner, if the weather is above freezing). They will need shelter and protection from other animals. A wind-proof dog house and a fenced yard are ideal.

Now is the time to find homes for those special pups. If they are registered, you will probably be able to sell them. But if they are of mixed ancestry, you will probably just have to exchange each pup for the assurance that it is getting a good home. Don't keep the pups so long out of love that you have trouble placing them. We have had terrific luck placing pups at a young age—but that "luck" severely diminishes when they become gangly and lose their cuteness (three to six months).

At six weeks, the pups should be wormed. Take a stool sample to your veterinarian to find out for sure if the pups have worms—and which kind they do have. (There are many types, all requiring different combinations of wormers.)

At eight weeks, the pups should be wormed again with the same wormer and receive their first adult distemper shot. This injection often includes protection against two other common dog diseases, leptospirosis and hepatitis. A booster is usually given about three months later, with a yearly booster necessary for complete protection. There is no one "permanent" shot.

A rabies shot is usually given at about six months.

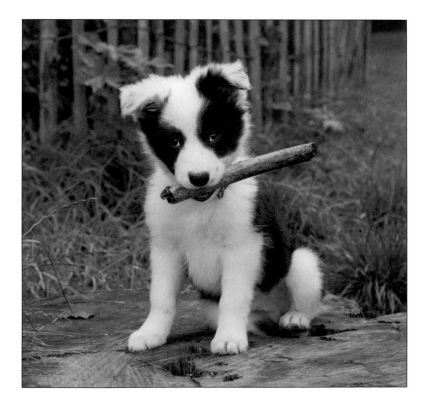

Kittens

KITTENS PROBABLY RANK next to pups in the numbers of domestic animal babies hand-raised by man. Cats also have litters, and there are a lot of cats—and cat lovers. Therefore, the odds again point to a greater chance of a person's encountering an instance where a kitten (or kittens) needs to be hand-raised.

THE ORPHANED, REJECTED, OR "NEEDY" KITTEN

There are many reasons why a kitten might need to be hand-raised. Perhaps the mother has died or is too weak or sick to nurse the kittens; maybe she has no milk or has an infection that prevents her from raising them safely. Occasionally a queen (correct term for female cat) rejects a kitten for some unknown reason.

Often there are three or more kittens in the nest, only a few days old—and you are their only chance for survival. So into a box they go! Be sure the kittens are warm enough in their box; provide heat if necessary to keep them comfortable.

Kittens are easiest raised if they nurse on a doll bottle with a rubber nipple or one of the pet nurser bottles sold at pet shops. Kittens, unless very weak, fight the feeding tube, so it is best not to use this method unless all else fails. (Maybe it's just that cats do not like to be rushed, even at that early an age!)

Most kittens will take about 8 cc of milk or more every two hours. We are partial to goat milk, but people have had good luck with commercial kitten formulas, and even human baby formulas in a pinch. Until they are about two weeks old, kittens should have their milk warmed to body temperature and kept there during feeding. If it

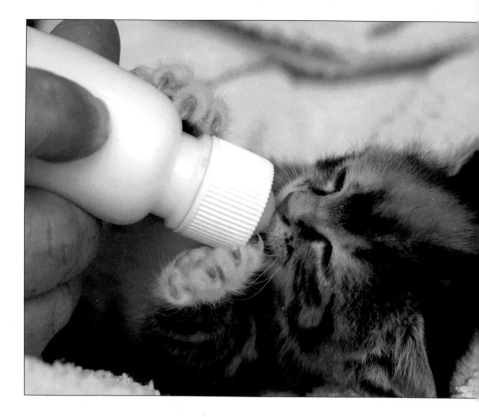

takes too long to feed the kittens, you may have to reheat the bottle by placing it in a pan of hot water. Take care to check the temperature of the bottle via the old drop-on-the-wrist method before giving it to a kitten, as the milk may have gotten too hot. You wouldn't want to burn a kitten's mouth.

Feed the kitten enough to satisfy it, but not enough to make it stop eating on its own. That is overfull. The kitten should look nice and round after feeding, but should not have a stuffed, hard, shiny belly.

After each feeding, massage the rectal area with a warm, damp washcloth. This will encourage elimination, and clean the kitten at the same time. Without this stimulation, kittens cannot eliminate properly and can become toxic. This must be done regularly for at least the first two weeks of life.

Kittens must be fed and cleaned up every two hours, day and night for two weeks. At this time you can safely add an hour between feedings, making only 8 feedings a day, instead of 12.

Keep the kittens in a smallish box, lined with a cake pan, covered with one or two towels, with a heating pad tucked safely underneath the towels. A towel may be draped over the top of the box, if there are any drafts in the area.

Do not handle the kittens, except at feeding time. Do not let small children handle them at all. Many kittens die from over-handling, even when they are six or eight weeks old.

WEANING FORMULAS

After the kitten is two weeks old, you can begin adding small amounts of high-protein infant cereal to the milk. This can gradually be increased until the gruel is thick enough so that the hole in the bottle must be slightly enlarged.

By three weeks of age, the kittens will probably lick small amounts of ground liver or kidney from your fingertip. At first their attempts will be messy and quite unsuccessful, but they will gain experience and, by six weeks, they will be able to eat all of their food from a dish.

FEEDING SCHEDULE: BIRTH THROUGH WEANING

	Birth to 2 weeks	2 to 4 weeks	4 to 6 weeks	6 weeks on
Milk	x	x	x	x
Hi-protein dry cereal	x	x	x	...
Ground liver/ kidney	...	x	x	x
Dry kitten formula/chow	...	...	x	x
Feedings per day	12	8	6	3

SYMPTOMS OF TROUBLE— AND WHAT TO DO

DIARRHEA

Diarrhea kills many hand-raised kittens, mostly because many people do not realize how deadly it is.

Milk can be irritating to the digestive system, especially when too large an amount is fed at one time. Therefore, take care not to overfeed the kittens, or to give them more milk at one feeding than they are used to having. When it is time to increase the amount of milk fed, do it very gradually, never more than 1 cc a day. The same goes for formula changes. If a formula must be switched, do it gradually, unless you have reason to believe that the kittens are allergic to the formula originally being fed.

Diarrhea kills kittens by dehydration and electrolyte imbalances. There is nothing mysterious about electrolytes. They are simply the normal body salts and chemicals. When a kitten has prolonged diarrhea, it loses not only body fluids during dehydration, but these body salts and chemicals as well. When this condition is prolonged, the organs do not function properly, and the kitten cannot live.

Never continue feeding milk to kittens with prolonged diarrhea. It will only irritate the intestinal tract, and little will be absorbed. If kittens have simple diarrhea caused by indigestion or overfeeding, just cut the next feeding in half, substituting warm water for the other half of the milk. If this does not solve the problem, give the kitten one-third of the amount fed of kaolin-pectin (with neomycin, if possible). (If you are feeding the kitten 9 cc of milk every two hours, give it 3 cc of kaolin-pectin every two hours, with the milk-water combination every other hour. This should clear it up within two feedings.)

Should the diarrhea be more severe and not clear up, discontinue feeding *all* milk, and replace it with the same amount of oral electrolyte solution. This will help the kitten combat the dehydration and electrolyte imbalance, and keep the bowels from receiving more irritating milk. Continue the kaolin-pectin every two hours, until relief is noted.

Should the diarrhea continue over 12 hours, even with treatment, contact your veterinarian.

CONSTIPATION

Constipation is fairly common in kittens and, like diarrhea, it can quickly kill them unless promptly treated. If a close record is kept of each kitten's elimination, there should be no problem in determining when a kitten might be constipated. Most kittens are quite regular. If the kitten passes two feedings and still has not had a bowel movement, though it did so previously, consider the possibility of constipation and watch the kitten carefully. It should not appear full before a feeding, nor the least bit listless. Should either of these conditions occur, along with the absence of bowel movements at feeding/cleanup time, give the kitten a warm, soapy enema. Give as much enema solution as half the amount normally fed, or until results are noted. An eye dropper works quite well on most kittens, but anything small enough, with a smooth tip will do.

Generally, this will quickly provide relief; the kitten will lose its potbelly and become more active.

Do not put off giving the enema. A kitten can be constipated as little as half a day and die from the toxins absorbed.

URINE BURN

Kittens seem prone to getting urine burn. This is a soreness of the genitals, similar to diaper rash in human babies, caused by contact with urine. The first sign of this will be a very red-looking rectal area. If let go, the area will swell and become so sore that the kitten will be reluctant to eliminate.

At the first sign of redness, wash the area well with warm water, drying it carefully afterward. Then apply some mild baby lotion. Do not use baby powder, as the talc in it may cause respiratory irritation and infection.

Be watchful of every kitten at each feeding, so that they are cleaned up very well and not allowed to become wet from urine in between feedings.

GENERAL CARE

Kittens are among the easiest babies to care for, once they reach weaning age. They may be kept either in the house or in an outbuilding, provided that the weather is suitable. If they are kept in the house, you can begin litter training them at six weeks. Kittens are creatures of habit where their toilet usage is concerned. Once they learn that the litter box is the place to "go," they will not use another place—*unless* another cat uses their box, or the litter box becomes foul due to infrequent cleaning.

After feeding, place the kittens—one at a time—in a fresh litter tray. They are used to eliminating after meals and will probably sniff around and finally use the box. Praise each one highly and return it to the nest box. Keep the litter tray clean, but do not overclean it at first, as kittens learn what the litter box is both by habit *and* by smell. Remember, though, that kittens have a greater sense of smell than we humans do, so don't let the box get so dirty that *you* can smell it. That might be "too much" for the kittens.

At eight weeks of age, the kittens should receive their vaccination for feline distemper (feline panleucopenia). While visiting your veterinarian for this vaccination, ask him his opinion on vaccinating the kittens for pneumonitis. In some areas, this is quite a problem in cats; in others, it is rarely seen.

Feline distemper, on the other hand, is quite common in cats, country-wide, and is often a quickly fatal disease. Treatment is frequently successful—if the disease is noticed in time. (Look for diarrhea, runny nose, and mattery eyes.) Seemingly healthy kittens can die from distemper in one day's time. Vaccination will prevent this possibility. After eight weeks of age, the kittens can be fed dry food free choice, with tidbits such as meat, canned cat food, and milk given a little at a time throughout the day. *Do not feed a lot of milk.* It does *not* cause worms, but it can cause diarrhea.

This is also the time to begin looking for homes for any kittens you do not plan to keep. After raising them all by hand, it is hard to think of these babies going to strange people. But it is better to have the kittens go to a home where they will be enjoyed and treated well, instead of having them stay with you, if you do not have the time or the money it takes (food, spaying, neutering, veterinary bills) to care for them or the room to house them properly. Cute little kittens are usually fairly easy to find good homes for, but it is very hard to find homes for half-grown cats—especially ones that have not been spayed or neutered.

At eight weeks, the kittens should also be examined for worms. This is done by your veterinarian. He can examine a small portion of fresh bowel movement under his microscope for the presence of worm eggs or larvae. Many kittens are infested with worms, so it is probable that your kittens will have some type of internal parasite. Your veterinarian will prescribe the correct worm medicine for the type of worm your kittens have. (Be aware that there are many, many types of worms infecting kittens.) *Do not just buy any worm medicine at the drugstore.* It will not get all types of worms and may be too toxic for your kittens. And if they do not have worms, there is no sense in giving them a toxic substance.

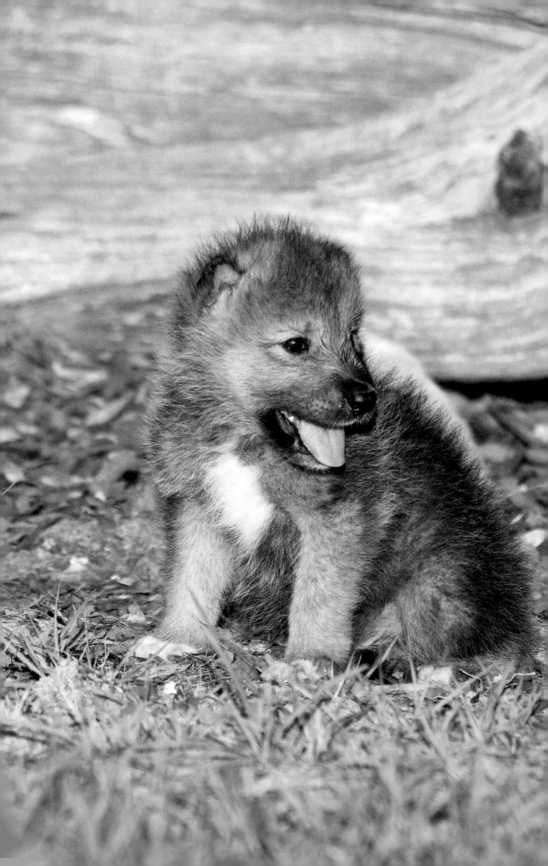

SECTION 2

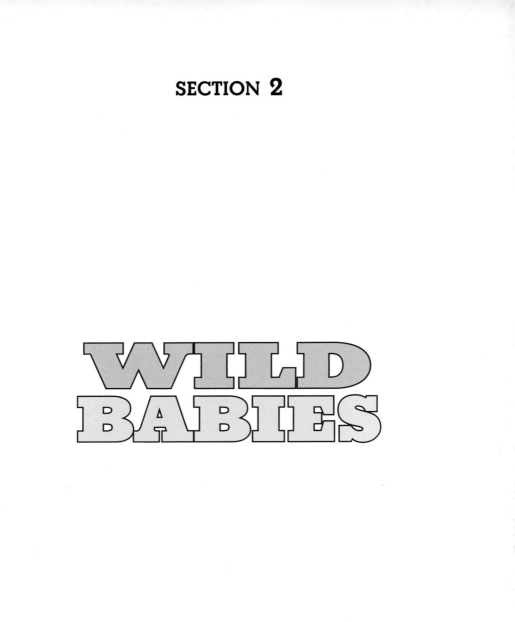

Wildlife Rehabilitation Centers or Licensed Breeders

Introduction to Wild Babies

THIS SECTION IS for licensed wildlife rehabilitators and licensed breeders of wild animals, including white-tailed deer, fox, coyotes, wolves, raccoons, bobcats, etc. State wildlife regulations forbid possession of wild animals (including orphaned or injured babies being raised for release) by unlicensed or non-permitted people. There are hefty fines involved for infringement of these laws, so please be very careful when you consider bringing that orphaned baby animal home to raise! In the first place, most "orphaned" wild baby animals are not really orphans at all. They are carefully hidden by their protective mothers while they go about daily life in the wild and are most likely very nearby, feeding and keeping watch over their baby. Some wild mothers are VERY protective of their young; it's best to watch from a distance to avoid disturbing a wild baby...and its mother! If you come upon a truly, verifiably wild orphan, it's best to keep it warm and call your veterinarian or game warden to find out where your nearest wildlife rehabilitation center is located and call them immediately.

Of course, there are many licensed breeders of wild animals who will occasionally be called upon to raise an orphaned or rejected baby, just like any farmer or breeder of domestic animals.

This section may also help zoo keepers who are called on to raise orphaned or rejected baby exotics. It matters not whether the "fawn" is a white-tailed deer or fallow deer, a cougar kitten or snow leopard. The basics are the same, and you will enjoy good results with good feeding and care.

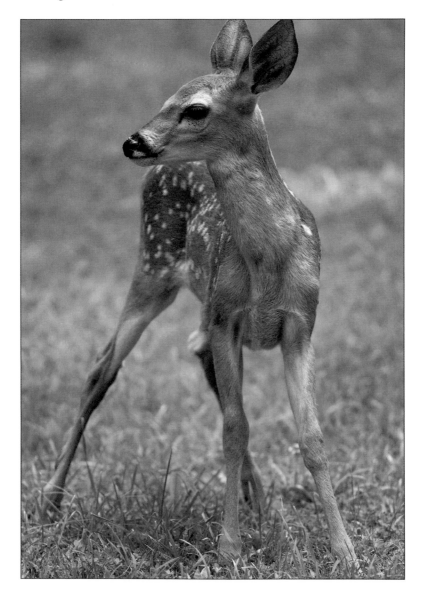

Fawns

THERE IS NO prettier baby, in our opinion, than the young fawn. This, coupled with Bambi stories and the high numbers of deer in fairly populated areas, makes the fawn high on the list of priorities in hand-raising wild babies. After all, most people would rather raise a fawn than, say, a baby mouse.

This likelihood can, and does, get a lot of fawns (and some people) into trouble.

ORPHAN FAWN OR HIDDEN FAWN?

In nature, the doe knows that her newborn fawn stands a much better chance of survival if it remains hidden in one spot, than it does if it follows her while she browses and goes for water. The fawn has very little body odor and very good camouflage patterns and colors on its coat. We've nearly stepped on fawns in the woods before seeing them and so have many hungry predators.

Unfortunately, many people who are unwise to the ways of wild animal mothers have found these hidden fawns and presumed them to be "abandoned" or "lost." Very, very, few fawns are abandoned or lost. These "found" fawns are, in effect, *stolen* from their mothers, taken home and handled, almost to death. They are fed indigestible

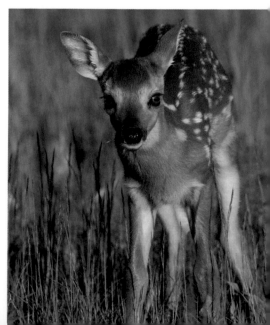

foods in too great quantities, but not frequently enough, and they soon weaken and die.

No wonder most areas have laws which prohibit the taking of protected wild animal babies—even to raise.

Before a fawn is removed from the wild, it is necessary to determine for sure whether or not the fawn is a true orphan. The only way to do this is to note the exact location of the fawn, perhaps marking a tree trunk near the fawn. The fawn should be left in that location, without being touched, overnight. If it is still in that place and shows evidence of not having eaten (it will appear more gaunt) you can safely assume that the fawn is an orphan.

When making the decision to remove the fawn from the wild, take into consideration the responsibility of rearing, and the many sleepless nights involved. The fawn will need feeding every two hours, day and night for at least a week, if it is a newborn.

Then consider the legality of what you are doing. In some areas, you need only contact the local game warden and he will readily give permission to keep the fawn long enough to raise it for release. We once lived in a place where the local game warden even brought us fawns discovered by other people who felt they were incapable of caring for them. We could raise the fawns until they were old enough to be on their own, and we would help them adjust to the wild life, finally freeing them entirely. In other areas, though, game wardens are very strict, not allowing anyone to raise a fawn or any other wild, protected baby. Where we live now, we are not allowed, legally, to keep even an injured fawn long enough to get it started right. Whatever the reason, you should become familiar with the game laws in your area, and be fully aware of the possible legal consequences of your taking on an orphan fawn to raise. Sometimes there is a fine of several hundred dollars involved.

It is important to determine the approximate age of the fawn so you can reasonably estimate the amount and frequency of feedings needed. All spotted fawns are not newborns! A fawn often carries spots into its second spring. A newborn fawn is very small, often weighing as little as 12 pounds. When it is very new, you will notice that the fawn has a damp umbilical cord and its hooves are quite soft. A few days after birth, the umbilical cord dries, but usually it is still hanging beneath the fawn's abdomen. The hooves have become black and hard. A three-week-old fawn can run quite well and is beginning to gain both size and strength. When you pick up a fawn of this age, do so with extreme care, as it can kick very hard with its tiny, sharp feet. Fawns do *not* like being restrained or picked up and will scream, kick, and fight to be put down.

A month-old fawn is a good armful, weighing, in many cases, 20 to 25 pounds. (Keep in mind, that there are several species of deer in the United States, from the small key deer in Florida, to the large mule deer in the western United States.) Larger fawns are dangerous to pick up. In their fright, they can seriously injure a person. If you are determined to try, it is best to have help, and to grasp the fawn firmly just under the throat, above the front legs, and just under the buttocks, above the hocks, and hold on tightly all around the fawn. Be prepared for thrashing, and keep your face turned away. If you can throw a coat over the fawn's head, it will calm down faster.

Be very careful in taking even a very young fawn home in the cab of your pickup or car seat. A frightened fawn can suddenly break free and leap through a closed window, or cause an accident by leaping onto your lap while you are driving. Try to have a helper along. Lacking a helper, don't try to tie the fawn's legs. Not only might you break one of its legs, but the fawn will probably thrash free anyway and injure itself or someone in the car.

A large burlap sack is the safest method of transporting a fawn. Place all four legs and the body in the sack, and allow the head to stick out. Close the sack snugly, but not too tightly. A good way is to cut a small hole, just large enough to admit the head, and tie the sack closed entirely. Don't let the hole get too large, or the front feet will soon follow the head and the fawn will wriggle free. A coat laid over the head will help if the fawn becomes agitated, due to being restrained by the bag. Don't let it bang its head on the floor of the car.

If at all possible, have a closet without windows, or a closed-in box stall in the barn to use as the fawn's pen, once it is brought home. Not only will this protect the fawn from accidents, but it will also help calm the animal.

Deposit the fawn in some clean bedding and leave it alone for a while to calm down and rest from its ordeal.

As the fawn rests, you can make arrangements for milk and other necessities for it. The best and easiest way to raise a fawn for release is to get a decent milking doe goat to act as a foster mother. With a little training, the fawn will be able to nurse off the doe goat. (See "Training the Nurse Doe" in the chapter *Kids*.) You may have to hold the doe so the fawn can nurse, but that sure beats filling and washing bottles—and the fawn has the added moral support of a like animal for company.

If the fawn is very new, try to feed some goat colostrum via the bottle, if necessary. This first milk is vital to provide some protection against disease during the fawn's first few weeks. It also provides a laxative to move the "stale" manure, which accumulated during the fawn's stay in the doe's uterus, from the bowels.

In general, the fawn can be treated like a kid goat. But take care not to make a pet out of the fawn, as it will probably have to be released to become a wild animal again. If the fawn becomes too tame, it will only get into serious trouble in the wild, and probably be killed.

THE INJURED FAWN

Quite often, the fawn that must be hand-raised has also been injured. Some of the most common injuries we have encountered include: dog or coyote bites, cuts from a hay mower, car accident injuries, near-drowning, fence cuts, and various hurts from animal traps. The first two account for about 75 percent of the injuries we have run across.

Some fawns that do have a mother nearby must still be taken in because their injuries are such that they could never follow their mother or survive in the wild. Broken legs are quite common, and they seldom, if ever, heal in nature. Most often, a predator finds the fawn in a weakened condition and kills it.

It is best, when bringing in an injured fawn, to take it to a veterinarian first thing. Some problems must have immediate attention. For example, sometimes a broken leg must be set at once to prevent permanent crippling or a necessary amputation.

You might note that we have had excellent luck using ketamine hydrochloride as an anaesthetic on fawns. This anaesthetic is not approved for use on other than cats and subhuman primates, but we have used it regularly for many years on deer and goats, with great success.

Broken legs can usually be pinned, which allows the fawn much greater freedom than if the leg has to be in a cast or splint.

When the injured fawn has been examined and treated by your veterinarian and then brought home, be sure to provide it with a very warm, totally enclosed pen for a week or two. Keep it there until the fawn is out of all danger from shock and has tamed down enough to be fed without a fight.

FORCE-FEEDING

It is quite possible that the wild fawn will neither nurse from the nurse doe nor a bottle fitted with a lamb nipple. Due to fear, very few fawns will just walk up and begin sucking on a bottle or nurse from a doe goat. But, of course, they must be fed, or weakness and death will surely follow.

There are two methods of force-feeding: tube-feeding, and forcing the nipple. (Tube-feeding is discussed in full in the chapter *Kids*, and the method used for fawns is exactly the same.) The fawn will have to be adequately restrained by a helper if necessary. We have gotten quite good results by just about sitting on the fawn (uninjured fawn), holding onto it with both of our hands and legs, and having a helper manipulate the nipple into its mouth. The fawn can usually be persuaded to taste the milk and then suck a little. Both tube-feeding and forced nipple-feeding are frustrating at first; but generally, the fawn begins to accept human help after two feedings and is willing to accept the bottle after three or four. As soon as the fawn accepts the bottle, discontinue the tube-feedings.

As soon as the fawn gains confidence and comes willingly for the bottle, it is time to introduce it to the goat's udder. Lure it to the doe's teat with the bottle, then coax it to trade the bottle nipple for the teat. Have a helper restrain the doe very carefully at first. Soon the fawn will come running when the doe is called! We had one fawn, Dotty, who thought *her* name was Rosie, the goat's name! We called "Rosie" and Dotty came flying, knowing it was feeding time. Even now, we can get Dotty to come to us in the woods by calling "Rosie."

FEEDING SCHEDULE: BIRTH THROUGH WEANING

	Birth to 1 week	2 to 3 weeks	3 to 5 weeks	5 to 8 weeks	8 weeks to 3 months
Milk	4 to 8 ounces	8 to 12 ounces	12 to 16 ounces	16 ounces	16 ounces
Feedings per day	12	8	8	6	4
Calf Manna	...	...	free choice	...	...
Mixed grain	...	...	free choice	...	...
Hay	...	...	free choice	...	...

If the fawn is nursing a doe goat, it will get the required amount automatically, as few fawns that are being fed every two hours from the doe will go hungry or overeat. Bottle-raised fawns can be fed, using this chart for a guide. Keep in mind that you will feed a fawn by size, not age. This can vary greatly, of course, so use your own judgment. Feed just enough to keep the edge off the fawn's hunger, keeping its sides full, but not bulging. Do not let it get so full that it rejects the nipple when offered.

SYMPTOMS OF TROUBLE— AND WHAT TO DO

DIARRHEA

Diarrhea is common in stressed fawns, especially those who have been hungry for a day or more, then are fed too much milk for the digestive tract to handle. The first few feedings must be fairly small to allow the fawn's digestive system time to handle milk again—especially milk that is entirely different from the kind it was accustomed to.

Prevention is the key to treating diarrhea. Fawns rarely starve to death due to being fed small amounts of milk very often—but many die from diarrhea, due to being fed too much.

Keep the fawn in a lightly bedded pen so that the droppings can be watched carefully. The young fawn's droppings are yellowish and a bit pasty, but formed. The week-old fawn's droppings are more goat-like, being well-formed and a dark color.

Should this consistency change toward the more fluid, cut the amount of milk being fed in half, and add half warm water in its place. If the diarrhea is caused by indigestion or simple overfeeding, it should stop immediately. If not, give from two to four ounces of kaolin-pectin (depending on the size and body weight of the fawn) every two hours, not at feeding time. This should quickly bring the diarrhea under control.

If the diarrhea does not stop, discontinue all milk, replacing it entirely with an oral electrolyte solution available at your drugstore or your veterinarian's office. Electrolytes are necessary in all cases of persistent diarrhea. When a fawn has diarrhea, it loses not only fluids, but also necessary body salts and chemicals as it dehydrates. These salts and chemicals are contained in the electrolyte solution and correct the electrolyte imbalance in the body, while replacing fluid. Milk really does neither at this point. Milk only serves to irritate the bowel further, worsening the diarrhea. Not enough is absorbed to provide nourishment or replace lost fluids.

Usually, the electrolytes, combined with the kaolin-pectin (with neomycin added if possible), will bring about quick relief.

If the diarrhea continues after more than 24 hours with treatment, call your veterinarian. The fawn may need parenteral (injected) electrolytes or additional antibiotics.

CONSTIPATION

Next to human stupidity and diarrhea, we would say that constipation kills more fawns than anything else.

The problem with constipation is that the fawn is often pretty far gone before the condition is noticed. It is not like diarrhea, with its often-messy symptoms which are easily noticed. There is no mess or smell with constipation. The active fawn all of a sudden acts tired and full. In fact, it even looks full. Well, it is full, but not full of fresh milk! If the fawn is not treated within a few hours of the time it first acts droopy, there is no chance of saving its life.

It is a very good practice to watch for droppings religiously, while observing the fawn. If no bowel movement is noticed and the fawn acts dumpy, suspect constipation at once.

When in doubt, give an enema. Fleet enemas, sold at the local drugstore for human babies, work very well on fawns. It is a good idea to keep one on hand—just in case.

Generally, an enema brings quick relief.

GENERAL CARE

One of the hardest things to do in raising a baby fawn is to control your desire to handle it and have it as a pet. You have to give it the best care possible, without letting it become too dependent on you—unless you really are able to keep it as a pet. Be cautious here, though. Even if you can legally keep the fawn, you may be in for trouble. You cannot fence a deer out of your flower beds, vegetable garden, or oat field. Nor can you keep it out of your neighbor's property. A deer does have wild instincts.

We dislike the saying that wild animals will "turn on" their owners. This is not true. But, wild animals, even pet deer *do* keep some of their wildness and *can* hurt a person who does not really understand them and their instincts. A wild animal is never really a pet, and a fawn will never act and react like a goat. It will always be a deer.

The safest place to keep the fawn is in a fenced area, with a wind-proof shelter for both the fawn and its foster mother, the doe goat. With company, the fawn should stay inside the fence, provided that the fence is made with the fawn in mind. The fence should be at least four feet high, and be either chain link or two-by-four-inch welded wire fabric. Stock fencing will not do, as the fawn will crawl through it and might run away or be attacked by ignorant children or a neighbor's dog.

Fresh water, hay, grain, and shelter are all the fawn will need until the time comes for its release.

It is a good idea, however, to have the fawn's droppings checked by your veterinarian for internal parasites. If some are found, the fawn should be wormed. Raised in domestic conditions, the fawn will be exposed to more parasites than if it were in the wild. After all, in the wild, fawns begin to browse here and there. They are not penned, but wander about and are not reinfecting themselves with parasites via contaminated feed and water.

TRAINING FOR RELEASE IN THE WILD

All the time you have the fawn, you must consider how everything you do is going to affect its eventual release. We have already discussed the inadvisability of making a pet of the fawn. This is but the first caution.

There are many things a person does that can hamper the animal's chances of survival after release. For example, we have seen people encouraging a friendship between a dog and the fawn. This may be novel and "cute," but it is also stupid. One of the greatest killers of deer in the wild is the dog. We don't mean only "wild" dogs, but the "bum" dog, the farm dog, and even the suburban pet poodle. We have seen all of these types chasing deer. The fawn that loses its fear of dogs will trust dogs in the wild, and possibly be killed by one.

Some people let everyone come to see the fawn they are raising and feed it tidbits by hand. This is also a bad idea, unless the fawn is heading for a park after release. Such a fawn will learn not to fear man and will calmly watch a hunter approach quite close. It may be against the law to hunt in a certain area or to hunt does, but you can be sure that there are some people who will hunt where they darned please, and who will kill anything that looks like a deer, no matter the sex or size.

SAFE RELEASE

There is no really "safe release" for a fawn, as there is no safety in the wild. But, there are a few things that can make the release and subsequent freedom as safe and free from fright as possible.

First of all, be sure to train the fawn for release from the time you begin to raise it. Then decide on the best place to release it.

Where we live now is the best place for us. We own 200 acres
bounded by deep swamp on two sides, with a neighbor across the road
with 600 acres of mixed open and woods. That also is bounded by
swamp. All the land is posted and we have very few trespassers. There
is good deer country nearby, with several small herds of deer within
two miles. There are few stray dogs.

All of our neighbors are sympathetic with our deer-raising and
keep an eye out for them after they are released. None have expensive crops that deer are likely to damage. When it is time to release
a grown fawn, we simply open the barn door and let the fawn come
and go at will. Usually it will venture about quite close to the barn
during the day but soon it will be seen roaming farther and farther
into the edges of the woods. Then, perhaps, one night it does not
come back to the barn. But the next morning it is back looking for
grain.

This will continue for some time, until the fawn finds deer
friends, or just decides to return to the wild. At this point, it may not
be seen for weeks at a time, and then will appear at the edge of the
woods—but it will seldom return, even for feed.

It is at this point that we feel good, even if it is painful not to have
the fawn trust us anymore. Now the fawn has been on its own and is
content with a deer's life, and is happy with things just as they are and
as nature intended them to be.

If you cannot release the fawn from your home, we think the best
way is to plan a camping trip in a remote area, preferably where hunting is not permitted. Notice that we do not say "release in the spring,"
or "release in the fall." Some fawns are able to survive a winter, and
others are not. This depends on several things. How severe is the
winter in your area? We live in northern Minnesota, with -50°F temperatures and a lot of snow. A small fawn cannot survive on its own
here. But, the same fawn could easily survive a Florida winter!

Release when the fawn is big and strong.

Do not free a fawn with a collar or harness on, thinking to protect it from hunters. Such fawns often die from strangulation after catching the collar or harness on brush.

If you can take the fawn and doe goat to your selected spot with some familiar feed, it will be best. Now, no fawn likes to ride, so the best thing is to have your veterinarian give it a tranquilizer which will last long enough to get the fawn to your camping spot. Once there, put up a small pen, just large enough for the fawn and goat. Unless the fawn and goat are penned for the first two days, the fawn will become terrified when it recovers from the tranquilizer and discovers it is in strange surroundings. It is likely to run off, probably never to return. It will be easier if the fawn can become accustomed to the area slowly, and without fright.

After two days' time, the fawn will usually settle down. It is then that the doe and fawn can be taken out of the pen. You can tie the doe near the pen, feeding the animals in the pen twice daily. The fawn will probably explore the nearby woods quickly, but will usually return several times. Be sure the area you have chosen is good deer country. It should have lots of young browse (such as willow, poplar, and aspen) and water available. With these conditions met, the fawn will just melt into the wild. If it remains gone for a day and night, you can pack up your gear and goat and head home. At first you will feel just terrible, but know that you have done the best you could for the fawn. Now it is grown and must be free to be happy.

Fox, Wolf, and Coyote Pups

ALL THREE OF these animals are basically wild dogs, and the whelping habits and care of the pups are basically the same as for dogs. All three build a nest in a den of some sort, in which to whelp their pups, with the fox generally digging a burrow deep into a hillside.

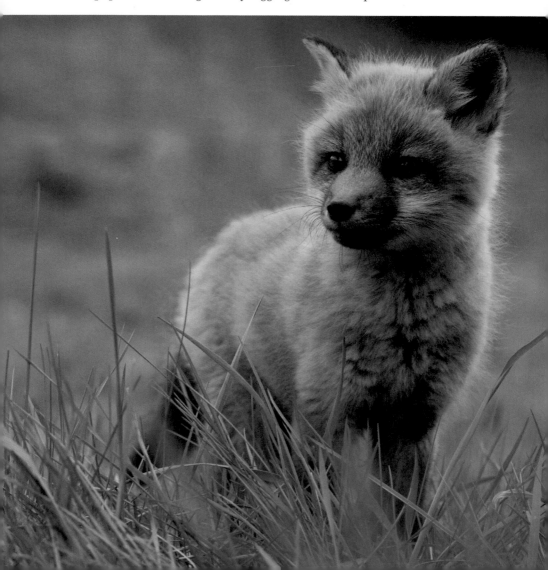

Not too many pups (from here on, we'll mean the young of the fox, wolf, or coyote when we say "pup") are seen at a young age. This is because their parents keep them well concealed in places seldom frequented by humans. Therefore, few people have the opportunity to raise the pups if they should be orphaned or injured. And, too, many people dislike and even hate the wild canines, due to their occasional preying on domestic animals. So, frequently, if pups are discovered, the finder's reaction is to destroy them as "enemies," not bring them home to raise.

THE ORPHANED PUP

Life in the wilderness can be dangerous and harsh. On occasion, a mother is killed while hunting to support her litter. If the pups are five or six weeks old (near weaning age), the father may be able to save them, as he often hunts for the family as well, bringing the kill home to the pups. They can survive without the mother's milk, although they would grow faster with it. But, when the pups are orphaned at a very young age (from birth to five weeks old), their chances of survival without human help are extremely slim.

Sometimes a person walking in the woods or fields comes across very young pups, obviously in need of help. We have found such pups, often with one or two dead in the den, and others nearby the den entrance.

These orphaned pups are very gaunt looking and usually quite weak.

Also, sometimes a person finds a dead female with enlarged breasts, showing signs of having nursed a litter of pups. This often happens on a road or highway where the mother has been struck by a car. Sometimes, if caring humans (and the orphaned pups) are lucky, they can search likely sites in the nearby vicinity and locate the den. But this is very hard to do, especially if you are not familiar with the habits of wild canines.

Young pups cannot live for more than 48 to 56 hours without nursing. Remember that in some areas, rabies in wildlife is fairly common. It is spread by saliva in scratches and bites. While it is not very commonly found in young wild canines, it CAN be a possibility. So take every precaution against being bitten or scratched, and if you should be, make sure you can identify the pup that injured you and contact your doctor when you get home, just to be safe.

Do not, however, bring home just any young pup or den of pups that you find. Many times, a pup or a litter is "stolen" from the den of a mother that is out hunting to become a "pet." This is *not* a good idea. First of all, it is illegal! It takes a lot of work to raise a young pup to adolescence. Wild canines also do not make good pets. They will not "turn on" you or any such garbage. But, they will keep their wild instincts intact—fighting to keep food, stealing from the trash bag, jumping on the table for food, marking their "territory" with urine and feces, and other un-pet-like behavior. Punishment does nothing but frighten the pup or make it angry. Few wild canines can be totally housebroken. And remember possession of a wild canine without a permit is illegal in most states.

A wild pup can be fun to raise—to adolescence—but very few people are equipped with the facilities, patience, and understanding to cope with the pup as he becomes an adult.

Be very careful when picking up orphaned pups after their eyes are open. These pups not only can see, but *bite* as well! And they will, too. Wear gloves if you decide to risk raising them. Rabies is common in wild canines, especially foxes. It is unlikely that the babies have been exposed but, should you be bitten, you may risk your life if you just ignore the fact that rabies is a possibility. Any time you are bitten by a wild baby that later dies, you should have it examined by a laboratory for rabies.

Otherwise, just be sure you are protected against tetanus.

THE INJURED PUP

Occasionally you may find, or have brought to you, a wild pup that has been injured. These pups are usually older pups, generally from five to eight weeks or older, as this is the time that they are beginning to venture from the den with or without their parents' "permission." And, as with all young creatures, they often get into difficult situations. Injuries range from dog bites, to broken legs, fence tears, and accidents on the road. Sometimes, a car will strike a mother and her litter, killing some, injuring the others.

Whatever the injury, *do not put yourself in the position of getting bitten!* Any animal can injure a person when the animal is in pain, but it is especially so with a wild animal that fears man to begin with. If an injured pup is found, try to work it into a sack or sturdy box carefully. Do not grab it by the body or you will aggravate any internal bleeding. An experienced person can quickly grab the pup by the scruff of the neck, quite close to the head, but we would not recommend this method for slow or easily frightened people. The pup usually shows every tooth in its head, while snarling and often urinating. If the person "chickens out," he or she usually gets bitten or injures the pup by dropping it.

As soon as the pup is in a warm, dark, safe place, it will usually quiet down and become easy to transport. Don't carry the pup close to your face, no matter how subdued it seems. We have a friend who rescued a pup from a trap and was carrying it in his arms to the truck when it suddenly revived and sunk its large, sharp canine teeth all the way through his nose and would not release its hold!

Take the injured pup to your veterinarian at once. After emergency treatment, be prepared to take the pup home for nursing.

Be sure to find out what the game laws are in your area regarding the fox, coyote, or wolf you have rescued. Should you disregard the game laws, be aware that you may be fined several hundred dollars for possession of the pup and that the game warden can take the pup from you, disposing of it in any way he decides is best.

FEEDING

Very young pups—those under two weeks old—have their eyes closed. These pups are usually quite safely handled and are best suited to tube-feeding for the first few days. (See the chapter *Pups* for directions.) Tube-feeding will allow them to become accustomed to being handled by humans. As with domestic puppies, wild pups should be fed every two hours, day and night. The amount fed depends on the species and body weight. Fox pups will generally take between 6 to 10 cc of milk, coyotes between 8 to 12 cc, and wolves between 10 to 20 cc. This is only a basic guide. The pups' abdomens should appear rounded after each feeding, but not bulging. If fed just right, they will gain weight and size steadily and not get diarrhea (the first sign of overfeeding).

They should be kept in a box lined with a cookie sheet (right side up), then several absorbent cloths, with a heating pad under the whole works. If it is cool in the house, you can drape a towel over the box.

After every feeding, each pup must be stimulated, by the use of a warm, damp cloth applied to the rectal area and abdomen, to eliminate. Without this stimulation, the pups will soon become toxic and die.

FEEDING SCHEDULE: BIRTH THROUGH WEANING

	Birth to 1 week	1 to 2 weeks	2 to 4 weeks	4 to 8 weeks	8 weeks on
Milk	x	x	x	x	...
Hi-protein dry cereal	...	...	x	x	...
Ground liver	...	...	x	x	...
Vitamin drops	x	x	x	x	x
Meat	...	...	...	...	x
Puppy formula dry dog food	...	...	...	x	x
Feedings per day	12	12	8	6	3

When the pups are comfortable during handling, try using a bottle in place of the feeding tube. The size of the bottle and nipple depends on the pups. Fox pups do best on a doll bottle with a rubber nipple or a pet nurser bottle, available at most pet shops. This is also true of very young coyotes. Older coyotes and wolf pups seem to like a human baby bottle with a smallish nipple. Begin feeding the same amount that the pup was getting via the stomach tube; then gradually, allow the pup to get *almost* as much as it wants. *Never* allow the pup to become entirely full as this may lead to indigestion.

As for formula, for the first two weeks we prefer using goat milk with a few drops of a good liquid puppy vitamin supplement added.

Then add a little high-protein baby cereal to each bottle of milk, gradually building up to a consistency just thin enough to go through an enlarged hole in the nipple.

SYMPTOMS OF TROUBLE— AND WHAT TO DO

DIARRHEA

Simple diarrhea is common in hand-raised pups. It is often caused by slight overfeeding, a change in the formula, or mild indigestion. Should one of the pups begin having loose stools, cut his milk in half, giving the other half in warm water. If this does not stop the diarrhea in two feedings, take a sample of the stool to your veterinarian for examination for internal parasites. Wild canine babies are often infected from before birth, or shortly thereafter, by internal parasites.

Worms and *coccidia* are quite common, generally affecting the pups only after they have been stressed. And it is quite a stress to be removed from a den after being hungry, changing formulas, and so on. If the pup's diarrhea seems to be caused by internal parasites, follow your veterinarian's recommendations as to worming or treating the coccidiosis.

If it turns out that it is just a severe case of simple diarrhea, you can usually stop it quite easily with treatment. First, give the pup half as much kaolin-pectin (preferably with neomycin added) as the amount of milk that you usually feed the pup, via feeding-tube or teaspoon. Smaller pups are easiest given medicine through the feeding-tube as they fight it less than the thick substance.

Repeat the kaolin-pectin (the neomycin will help treat any bacterial infection present in the digestive tract) treatment every two hours. In two treatments, the pup usually has stopped passing loose stools. If not, cut out all milk being fed, and replace it with oral electrolyte solution. As the pup continues with the diarrhea, it becomes dehydrated. In dehydration, the pup not only loses body fluids, but also necessary body salts and chemicals.

If milk is fed, it irritates the delicate membranes in the bowels even more, and it is so poorly absorbed that it contributes little to the needed fluids and electrolytes. The oral electrolyte solution is absorbed and does not irritate.

Generally, electrolytes coupled with kaolin-pectin (not given together, but every other hour), bring about a quick recovery.

You may feed the electrolytes in place of the milk for 24 hours, if necessary. After this time, if the pup still has loose stools, again contact your veterinarian. The pup might need injectable electrolytes, or additional antibiotic or sulfa treatment.

CONSTIPATION

Constipation is not often a problem in wild pups as they are generally very good eaters, which seems to keep them quite regular. Should a pup suddenly seem full *before* a feeding and act a little sleepy or dopey, suspect constipation at once.

An enema is quite easy to give a pup, and it generally brings quick relief. You can use any instrument that is small enough and has a smooth tip, and big enough to hold the correct amount of warm, soapy water. An infant ear syringe works well. The pup should be given half as much enema solution, rectally, as the amount of milk it is usually fed, or until desired results are seen.

FLEAS

Fleas are quite common on wild canines, but they can cause discomfort and even weakness in young pups. All pups should be inspected thoroughly at feeding time for tiny, quick-moving insects, especially on the head and back.

If any are noticed, dust all the pups with a rotenone insecticide. Do not use anything else on young pups, as there are many insecticides on the market that contain harsh and dangerous chemicals. There are often more warnings on such a box than directions!

WORMING

If the pups' stools have not been checked by your veterinarian for the presence of worm eggs, larvae, and *coccidia* (one-celled parasites), at six weeks of age this should be done. If your veterinarian finds evidence of any of these, he can prescribe the correct medication. Do not just buy some worm medicine at the drugstore and worm the pups. There are many types of worms, each requiring different drugs and combinations to deal with them effectively. It will do no good to use a drug that is either too mild to kill the worms that the pups have, or is so strong that it will kill the pups along with the worms!

GENERAL CARE

Care of the pups for the first three weeks of age is a painstaking, but easily followed routine: keep warm and dry, feed, stimulate, clean, and so forth.

As the pups reach 8 to 10 days of age, their eyes will be open, and they will start to take small bits of ground liver from your fingertips. At this age, they will also begin to toddle away from their "nest" to eliminate. The pups do not want to lie in their mess, so they will begin "house-training" themselves. Keep their box as clean and dry as possible. This is easiest done by having a long, deep box, such as a refrigerator box, with the nest in one end, and the "potty" in the other. The latter should be covered well with a thick layer of newspapers which should in turn be covered with a layer of wood shavings. Shredded newspapers also work, but they won't do much for the smell, which is inevitable. Coyote pups, especially, have a disagreeable odor, particularly when startled.

At five weeks, the pups will begin to tumble about, playing quite roughly with each other—and you. If they get too rough with you, do not slap them for they won't understand what you mean. Instead, discipline them as their mothers would have done: grab them by the back of the neck, give them a good shake, and hold the head down on the floor. This will bring about a submissive gesture from them—a grimace (which looks like a horrible snarl to the uninitiated), and possible urination. It will only take a time or two for the pups to learn just how hard they dare to bite you before you "bite." This punishment does not bring fear or hate, but just a deep respect, and an acceptance of you as their "pack member" superior.

If the weather permits, you can move the pups outdoors after six weeks, provided that they have a warm nest box or dog house to curl up in. They should also be provided with a strong, tight fence, at least six feet high. This will keep them from wandering off and protect them from stray dogs as well. A chain link or two-by-four-inch welded wire fence is easily erected and strong.

If the pups are being raised for release, as most should be, do not make pets of them. This will only reduce their chances of survival in the wild. If they trust man entirely, they will be in great danger from the time they are released.

The pups will maintain enough wild instincts, if they are exposed to few people and no other animals. It is a big temptation to make the pups act like little dog puppies—but remember they are not!

SAFE RELEASE TO THE WILD

If you are able to release two or more pups at the same time, things will go easier for them. They will have each other for moral support and help in hunting. The single pup will have it a bit harder, so it is best if it is released when it is a bit older. A litter of pups can be released at about 8 months of age and have a reasonably good chance of survival. The single pup should be held back until it is 10 months old.

If it is possible to do so prior to release, take the pups on several field trips—trips to the woods—and encourage them to hunt. Help them tip over logs and dig out mouse nests. Show them the edge of the marsh, where voles and frogs are common. Plan to spend several hours on each trip, all the while encouraging the pups to hunt for their lunch.

After several trips like this, the pups will be quite eager and ready to hunt for their livelihood.

Plan to spend a couple of days camping in the spot where you are to give the pups their final release. Choose the spot with care. Remember that wild canines can get into trouble by raiding farms. This is especially true of pups that have been hand-raised, so try to release them far from such temptations. Consult your game warden. Quite probably, he will be able to tell you of a very good spot, remote, and with good hunting for the pups. Take the pups there in a crate, along with a bag of dry dog food.

Plan to arrive in the late afternoon, not releasing the pups until the next morning. The reason for this is so that you can go along with them on their first day in the wild and be their "mother," giving them confidence to go ahead and hunt or play—in other words, giving them freedom to be natural.

You can feed them that night, if they did not have luck hunting, but try to get them to eat some prey, even if it is only a field mouse or a frog. Take them out again, but this time drop back, letting them go more and more on their own. If they roam out of your sight, do not follow.

Return to camp and try to relax. They may not return. If they do, don't pen them up, but let them be free at night. They may pester you all night, nibbling at your ears or tearing your sleeping bag, but they may decide to become wild ones, leaving you in the middle of the night.

When they do leave, you can pack up. We usually leave them dry dog food at the campsite in case of emergency: poor hunting.

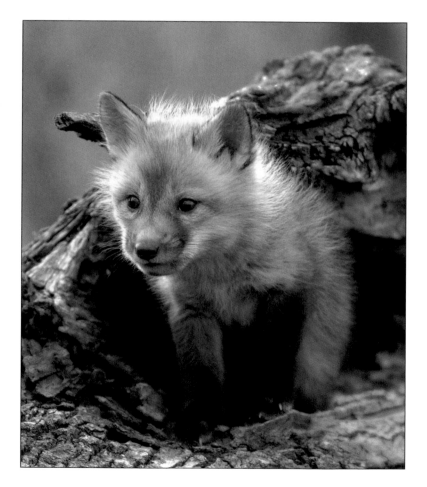

Bobcat and Cougar Kittens

VERY FEW PEOPLE have the opportunity to raise any of the native wild kittens. This is due, in part, to the relative scarcity of lynx, bobcats, and cougars, and in part to their secretive habits. Very few people ever see the young kittens of these cats, and only a small percentage of these people who glimpse the kittens will ever run across orphan kittens.

When kittens are found, a person should be *very* sure they are orphans before popping them into a sack to take home. Some mama cats are very protective of their young, even to the point of attacking a person who threatens them. (Remember, anything that causes the kittens to squall is "threatening" them, according to mama cat's instincts.)

THE ORPHANED KITTEN

Before picking up any wild kittens, a person has to check for signs that they really are orphans. If they have been without a mother for over a day, the kittens will have lost a lot of energy and body weight. Their abdomens will be gaunt, and they will act whiny and depressed. One or more of the kittens may be dying or dead. There are generally from one to four kittens in a litter, and it is generally the smaller kittens, or "runts," that perish first.

If the kittens have been orphaned very recently, they will have more spunk, depending on age, but will lose it in several hours if the mother does not return. It is best to feel the abdomens of the kittens, then go away for two or three hours (depending on the age of the kittens, of course—tiny kittens will be severely weakened in two hours time) and then return. If the mother has come back, she may

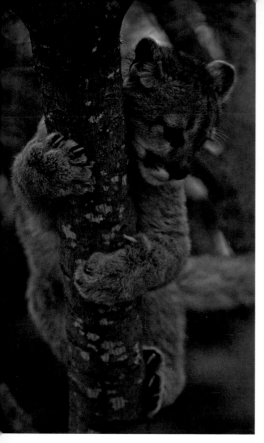

have moved the kittens to a "safer" place, where there is no human scent around, or she will have fed the kittens, whose abdomens will then feel more rounded and hard.

When you feel that you have a bunch of genuinely orphaned wild kittens, try to get them all safely into a sturdy sack or box for the trip home. If the kittens have their eyes open, they will be very frightened and appear like little devils, spitting and growling at a mere touch. They will also claw and bite, given the opportunity, so be careful to stay out of reach. Gloves will give a certain amount of protection, but four-week-old cougar kittens can nip through all but very heavy leather gloves.

Remember that in some areas, rabies in wildlife is fairly common. It is spread through saliva in scratches and bites. While it is not very commonly found in young wild felines, it CAN be a possibility, so take every precaution against being bitten or scratched, and if you should be, make sure you can identify the kitten that injured you and contact your doctor when you get home, just to be safe.

It's easiest to grasp baby kittens by the scruff of their neck, holding firmly so that they can not swing around. In this way, they will not be injured, and neither will you!

Before even taking the wild kittens home, you need to call your local game warden or wildlife rehabilitation center. It is illegal to possess wild felines, even to nurse them back to health and release them. There are stiff fines for infringement of these game laws, so without a license and permit, leave the raising of these babies to rehabilitators who have the experience to make a success of raising these orphans.

For those who can legally help orphaned or rejected wild felines, the following may help your effort succeed.

Young bobcat kittens will nurse best on a pet nurser bottle with rubber nipple or a large doll's bottle with a rubber nipple. Do not get a bottle with a plastic nipple, as the kittens will reject it and not get enough to eat. Older bobcat, lynx, and cougar kittens will do best on a human baby bottle.

We prefer goat milk as a substitute for "wild cat" milk, as it is easy to digest—much easier than cow milk. Many people have had luck with artificial formulas, made just for domestic cats.

It is also a good idea to add a few drops of a good multiple vitamin formula purchased from your veterinarian. Such vitamins are a great help in getting the kittens over the stress of changing formulas and being hungry for several hours, or days.

It is very important that the kittens be fed every two hours, day and night, if they are newly born. In fact, until the kittens' eyes are open at about 7 to 10 days of age, they will need these frequent feedings. The kittens' digestive tracts are geared to take small amounts at frequent intervals. When large amounts are fed, a kitten soon develops indigestion and diarrhea. If the kittens are not fed often enough, they will die. In fact, missing one feeding is often enough to kill a kitten!

As soon as the kittens are brought home, they should receive a feeding. There is no way to know how long they have gone without feeding, so it is important to get something into them at once. Sometimes these kittens are so frightened and upset by their close contact with strangers that they hiss and spit, not accepting the bottle at all. In this case, you must tube-feed them a time or two so that they will live long enough to calm down. (See the chapter *Pups* for detailed information on tube-feeding.) Getting a tube down the throat of a frightened kitten is not a simple matter, but it is necessary. So wrap the kitten up, have a helper hold it firmly, and work as gently as possible.

The amount of milk needed varies with the body weight and age of the different kittens. A bobcat kitten that is newly born will usually take from 12 to 20 cc of milk; a lynx kitten, from 15 to 25 cc; and a cougar kitten, about 20 to 25 cc. This amount will vary greatly, depending on the care the kittens received before you found them (some mothers give a lot of milk—others very little), the size of the individual kittens (the larger the litter the smaller the kittens, as a rule), and the area where the kittens were found.

Just be sure that the kittens get enough milk to make their abdomens look nice and plump, but not hard and bloated looking. If they are getting the right amount of milk, they will sleep well between feedings, moving their legs, twitching and mewing on occasion. If they are getting too much milk, they will quickly develop diarrhea. If they are not getting enough milk, they will mew constantly, look thin, and soon die if the amount is not increased.

As the kittens are fed, place them in a warm cardboard box, lined with a cookie sheet then several towels, and underneath the towels goes a heating pad.

Immediately after each kitten is fed, you must massage the abdomen and rectal area, which stimulates their elimination reflex. If this is not done, not only will the kittens soon be very messy, but they may become constipated or retain their urine, which causes them to become extremely toxic.

THE INJURED KITTEN

Kittens that are injured are usually older kittens, over six weeks of age. Before that time, they stay in the den or very close to it, and seldom run into trouble. Like children, as the kittens grow older they become far more adventuresome, often running into situations that can be dangerous. Falls from rocky ledges, dog bites, and injuries caused by male cats are common.

If a kitten can simply be rescued from its trouble and soon set free for the mother to take care of, it is best for the kitten. But, some injuries to kittens require veterinary assistance or extensive nursing. Such kittens would not survive in the wild and should be raised in a protected environment.

As with the orphaned kitten that is healthy, know your state's game laws concerning injured kittens, and contact your game warden for the phone number of the nearest wildlife rehab center.

FROM BOTTLE TO WEANING

As the kittens gain weight and size, they will begin drinking more and more milk. Always keep the "tummy gauge" in mind. (The kittens' abdomens should look nicely rounded after each feeding, but not grossly enlarged and shiny.)

As soon as the kittens' eyes open, you can begin adding a little dry, high-protein baby cereal to their milk. Keep giving the vitamin drops until the kittens are weaned. After they are three weeks old, you can add a little ground raw liver and mashed egg yolk (hard-boiled) to the cereal-milk combination, keeping the whole formula thin enough to pass through the hole in the nipple without a lot of enlarging.

Be a little careful when feeding the kittens after they reach five weeks, as they may be a little hungry after the feeding and become a bit resentful when you take the bottle away. Resentful kittens can bite and scratch!

At five weeks, you can begin offering them a little of the cereal-milk-liver-egg, thickened a bit, from the end of a teaspoon. The fingertip can be used, but sometimes a hungry kitten will not only lick the food from the finger, but grab the hand, while "protecting" the food he has found. And, those needle sharp claws do dig in.

WEANING

When the kittens are almost entirely weaned, which happens at eight to nine weeks of age with most kittens, they should be receiving both milk and a mixture of high-protein dry cereal and ground liver in their bottle. Remember the added vitamins as well.

The kittens should also be taking a fair amount of this formula, in a thicker consistency, from a shallow pan. At about eight weeks, the kittens will be able to handle some additional meat. This should be chopped in fairly small pieces (about the size of the end of your thumb) until the kittens get used to chewing larger pieces. At first they will snatch a large piece, then try to quickly gulp it down, possibly choking on it. A good way to teach a *kitten* to chew is to give it a *large bone* with some *meat attached*. Here, it will have to gnaw and lick the meat to get at it with no danger of choking.

As the kitten begins eating this meat, it is a very good idea to sprinkle it with a tablespoon of cod-liver oil, then roll it in a tablespoonful of bonemeal. You can get both from your local feed dealer at a much lower price than from a drugstore, and you'll be buying both in a greater quantity than you would from a drugstore. Each kitten should receive one feeding that has been fortified with the cod-liver oil and bonemeal daily to be sure it gets adequate vitamin D and calcium. Many hand-raised kittens suffer from rickets, due to being fed only the muscle part of the meat and spending a lot of time in a cage or indoors. In the wild, kittens at weaning age, and even before, spend a great deal of time out of the den and, when they are fed by the mother, they eat not only muscle meat, but intestines, body organs, bone and some intestinal contents.

SYMPTOMS OF TROUBLE— AND WHAT TO DO

DIARRHEA

Simple diarrhea is common in hand-raised kittens. It often shows up about three days after the kittens have been in the home. Usually, it is due to the kittens' having been hungry for a period of time, then receiving a feeding of a formula foreign to them along with the stress of being handled by humans.

If, at the first sign of diarrhea, the amount of milk being fed is cut in half, with the missing half being substituted by warm water, the problem usually clears right up. If not, give the kittens half as much kaolin-pectin (with neomycin added, if possible), as the milk usually fed, every two hours, in between feedings of milk-water. This usually clears the problem up within four hours.

FEEDING SCHEDULE: BIRTH THROUGH WEANING

	Birth to 2 weeks	2 to 3 weeks	3 to 5 weeks	5 to 8 weeks	8 weeks on
Milk	x	x	x	x	...
Hi-protein dry cereal	...	x	x	x	...
Ground liver	...	...	x	x	...
Vitamin drops	x	x	x	x	x
Chopped meat	...	...	...	x	x
Feedings per day	12	12	8	6	4

If not, cut out all milk being fed. Milk is irritating to the digestive tract and if it is continued past this point, it won't help, but will do harm by keeping the bowels irritated and worsening the diarrhea.

As diarrhea progresses, the kitten becomes dehydrated to some extent. As this dehydration occurs, the kitten not only loses body fluids, but also body salts and chemicals, known as electrolytes.

Now, not only must fluid be given, but also a solution of electrolytes. A ready-made electrolyte solution can be purchased from any drugstore (they sell it for human babies with diarrhea) or veterinarian. This solution should be given in the place of milk being fed. Completely replace the milk-water solution with electrolytes. Give as a regular feeding every two hours, with the kaolin-pectin-neomycin between times, every hour.

If this treatment does not bring relief in 12 hours (little kittens) to 24 hours (big kittens), call your veterinarian. The kittens may need injectable electrolyte treatment or additional antibiotics.

CONSTIPATION

Constipation is generally only a problem with wild kittens for the first week you have them in the home. (However, you must massage the abdomen and rectal area after every feeding, until the kittens are able to crawl about.) We have found that when you get the kittens on a regular feeding schedule, they seldom have any problem with constipation.

A constipated kitten is usually in trouble fast. It may eat well at one feeding, but not pass a bowel movement. At the next feeding it may only eat a little, then reject the nipple. At the next feeding it will appear cold and very depressed. Soon it will be dead.

The constipation must be caught early. If it is not caught by the time the coldness and depression set in, there is little chance to reverse the outcome. Kittens generally pass a stool after each feeding. Note each kitten's routine. If one skips, note that also, and carefully check it at the next feeding. If it does not seem hungry and the abdomen appears full, but soft, strongly suspect constipation.

You can give an enema with a child's ear syringe, or anything with a smooth tip that will hold enough warm soapy water for the enema.

You will need as much water as half of a regular feeding, as a rule—or give a little at a time, until results are obtained.

SCRATCHING

Some litters of young wild kittens are bothered by scratches given to each other as attempts are made to nurse on each other. Little sores on the belly and face will tell of this problem. If this happens, simply clip the sharp hook off the nails on each kitten. If just the tip is taken, it will neither hurt nor bleed, nor will it harm the kitten for future release, as it will grow back.

URINE BURN

Occasionally, urine burn becomes a problem. You will notice this as redness in the genital area, sometimes accompanied by swelling. It is similar to diaper rash in human babies and is treated similarly. Keep the kittens clean and dry at all times. If they are wetting in between feedings, use a disposable diaper under them to absorb any drops of urine, and this will prevent the kittens from coming into contact with the irritant.

At eight weeks, take a small sample of stool to the veterinarian for a worm check. If the kittens do have any type of internal parasite, the veterinarian will be able to prescribe the correct medicine.

Use a mild baby lotion on the kittens' raw spots. *Do not* use baby powder, as the kittens may develop an allergic disorder from breathing in the dust. Powder is fine for human babies who have a foot or more between one end and the other. But the opposite ends of kittens are separated by only a few inches—and the talcum does fly around a lot.

GENERAL CARE

Remember that it is usually illegal to possess any wild baby animals, even if you mean well and only mean to raise them to release into the wild. Contact your local game warden for the name and phone number of the nearest wildlife rehabilitation center.

If you are licensed and permitted to raise baby wild animals, the following information may help you raise your babies successfully.

The kittens will have to be kept in a pen until they are old enough to survive in the wild, about age eight months. Whenever possible, we really believe it is best to keep the kittens until after they are a year old. Though eight-month-old kittens are able to hunt, they will not have an established territory as winter comes on.

If it is not possible to keep them through the entire winter, it is best to release them at eight months, so they will have at least a two-month period to establish a territory and learn how to hunt before severe winter sets in.

If the kittens are going to be held until they can be released in the spring, they will need a more permanent pen. As their strength and curiosity grow, they will soon tear holes in welded wire pens and chicken wire. A six-foot-high chain link fence enclosure with a chain link roof will be needed. The growing kittens will need a larger area to roam. Allow 50 square feet per kitten. It is a good idea to place a sturdy log inside to encourage healthy rough and tumble activity.

If you live in a remote area, take the kittens with you for jaunts in the field or woods. This will be the most important part of their juvenile period, as they will, bit by bit, learn to hunt. Take care, however, that the kittens (now looking more like adults) don't get near other people or farm animals. Panics are started this way! After all, how many old ladies, weeding a garden, are prepared for the sight of three cougars galloping across the lawn?

All the time you have the kittens, you will have to keep in mind that they are wild, potentially dangerous animals, no matter how tame and affectionate they seem. If they didn't have these instincts, they could never survive in the wild. The kittens may be very protective of their "kill" (even if it is a bowl of chopped meat and dry cat food). They may become very angry if you try to remove them from the couch or waste basket. And they may play very rough with you, not realizing that your skin is not as tough as theirs. You will not be able to punish these kittens, so don't try. Any attempt (other than very mild smacks with a rolled-up newspaper) will cause angry or fearful responses from the kittens.

As long as the kittens are in captivity, you should supplement their diet with cod-liver oil and bonemeal. You should also try to get them some meat other than liver or muscle meat. A good source is a local slaughter house. Beef scraps, such as stomach, tripe, lungs, kidneys, and bruised areas, will not only give the kittens a good variety of meat, but also help cut down on the budget. It does cost quite a bit to buy meat "over-the-counter" for three cougar teenagers.

Do not feed dry dog food to save money on meat. It is not high enough in protein for the kittens, and they will not do well on it.

We believe that the best thing the average foster parent of wild kittens can do is to raise the kittens with release in mind, so their ultimate way of life can be fairly easy for them. The kittens should not be handled often by anyone other than the family that is raising them, and the handling done by them should be limited to feeding, cleaning (well maybe just a *little* playtime!), and moving them from place to place.

Visitors to the kittens should not be allowed to play with them. The more people that the kittens see and trust, the more chance there will be for them to come to a bad end from trusting the wrong person when they are free—a hunter, for example.

The kittens should not be allowed to play with a dog. This will make the kitten believe that dogs can be trusted—a deadly belief in the wild.

The kittens should not be played with as though they were domestic kittens, by offering the hand to pounce on. As a playful adult, the "kitten" may stalk and "pounce" on a person, scaring him to death, and causing the cat to be hunted down as a killer.

SAFE RELEASE TO THE WILD

It is best to plan a vacation, if possible, at the same time you plan to release the kittens. They often need two weeks' time, or more, to establish a territory. In establishing a territory, they will need to learn to hunt, where the best hunting is, where and what possible enemies there are, where safe water is and where safe sleeping areas are to be found. The first four days in a new territory, the kittens will probably slink around low to the ground, jumping at every new sight. Try to take them to a pond's edge, where small animals and frogs are found in abundance. It is unreal to expect them immediately to be able to kill a rabbit or deer, as their hunting skills are about zero, unless you have been giving them some training previously. If they catch a field mouse or vole, or even a frog, they will be doing well.

If the area is remote enough, once the kittens relax a bit and begin to hunt, their biggest problems will be over. Man is the biggest enemy of wild cats.

Generally, after two weeks' time, the kittens will be on their way to being little hunters, provided that you really train them—and don't give them a good feeding because you feel sorry for them. You will have to live, more or less, like a wild animal with them, taking the kittens through brush and woods (take a compass, and don't get lost), and over rocks and gullies.

Once they feel secure, the kittens will begin drifting farther and farther away from you. At this point, let them go.

Raccoons and Opossums

RACCOONS AND OPOSSUMS are quite common in most areas of the United States and are found in close proximity to humans. Both, in fact, seem to enjoy people—or maybe it's their garbage cans that the animals enjoy! Both are "cute" babies, often being found and hand-raised by people. Both animals are scavengers of a sort, commonly seen on roadsides, looking for "goodies" thrown out of cars, small dead animals, and so forth. Unfortunately, the babies often accompany the mothers at a young age (especially in the case of the opossum, where the babies are in the pouch). Many times, a car will strike a mother on one of her foraging missions, killing her and several babies. The survivors need human assistance or they cannot live.

THE ORPHAN

When young raccoons and opossums are found, it is first important to be sure they are orphans. If young raccoons are found in a hollow tree or other "nest" and appear full of milk and are active, they are probably being cared for by a very live mother. If, on the other hand, they are a bit listless, gaunt, or if you have found the mother dead, you will be quite sure that the babies need help.

If the mother has been dead for several hours, the babies will be very hungry, acting hyperactive. If she has been dead for 12 hours, the babies will be nearly starved to death—if not so. They will feel cold, be quiet and still. When these babies are found, it is usually best to get them warm quickly. If they must be carried any distance, put them in an inside pocket, next to your body, or on a sun-warmed car seat.

Remember that in some areas, rabies in wildlife is fairly common. It is spread by saliva in scratches and bites. While it is not very commonly found in young wild raccoons and opossums, it CAN be a possibility, so take every precaution against being bitten or scratched, and if you should be, make sure you can identify the animal that injured you, and contact your doctor when you get home, just to be safe.

As soon as possible, get some warm Karo syrup and water (mixed half and half) into them. If they will take the mixture from an eye-dropper, fine. If not, use a feeding tube (a much smaller size than used for larger babies), as described in the chapter *Pups*. Do not feed milk to these babies yet. It will not be digested, and they need the sugar and energy *right now*.

Next, it is important to figure out how old the babies are, in order to feed them correctly. (See illustrations.)

Raccoons develop similarly to puppies and kittens. Their eyes don't open until they are 20 to 23 days old. But, opossums are another story. At birth, they are about the size of a kidney bean, naked and hairless. They move to the mother's pouch, where they stay for about two months, nursing almost constantly. At about two months of age, they develop hair, and their eyes open. It is during this period that they venture from the pouch and ride on the back and belly of the mother, returning to the pouch to nurse.

It is very difficult to raise naked, blind baby opossums. We believe this is partly due to the fact that they require very small, nearly constant feedings, and are very delicate.

Both baby opossums and raccoons are easiest raised on a doll bottle or pet nurser with a smallish nipple (rubber, of course, not hard plastic). Do not use an eyedropper, or you may give them too much formula at once and cause them to inhale milk droplets. This often kills them, due to inhalation pneumonia.

After giving the new babies their first feeding of Karo syrup and water, place them in a warm cardboard box. The box must be kept warm with either a heat lamp or a heating pad, placed under the box, and protected from dampness by a cookie or cake pan.

Remember that it is usually illegal to possess any wild baby animals, even if you mean well and only want to raise them for release into the wild. Contact your local game warden for the name and phone number of the nearest wilflife rehabilitation center.

If you are licensed and permitted to raise baby wild animals, the following information may help you raise your babies successfully.

Also, in some locations, it is even illegal to release a raccoon or opossum into the wild because of the possibility of them being infected with rabies. Be sure you are legal!

This warmth and frequent small feedings are the essentials of raising these babies. We prefer to use whole, raw goat milk, as a substitute for the mother's milk. Other people have used Esbilac or the human baby formula Enfamil. It is best to pick one and stay with it, unless the babies obviously cannot handle the formula.

After each feeding, the babies should be stimulated to eliminate. This is done by massaging the abdomen and rectal area with a warm, damp cloth. Without this stimulation, they may hold their urine and feces, becoming toxic from the waste materials.

The babies must be fed every two hours, day and night, when quite small. Raccoons need this every-two-hour feeding schedule from birth to three weeks. Opossums, which are really undeveloped fetuses when "born," need these frequent feedings from the time they are born to the age of two-and-a-half months.

Allow the babies to have *almost* as much milk as they want at each feeding. Never let them get entirely full. Stuffed babies usually die, due to indigestion and diarrhea.

WEANING FORMULAS

RACCOON

Baby raccoons will start experimenting with a little food other than their bottle formula at about four or five weeks. You can start with solid foods, such as the dry baby cereals and vegetables and meat that have been put through a blender and added to the milk, even sooner. Just keep the whole formula thin enough to go through the bottle's nipple. And remember that all food changes and additions must be made *slowly*.

At first the baby raccoons will pat and play with the food offered, rather than gobble it down. But soon they will nibble a bit at it in their play and decide that they like their new toy—to eat!

A good-quality canned dog food or cat food is a good starter food for baby raccoons. Don't bother with the cheaper foods, containing mostly cereal—you are already feeding him that. And, don't bother with the kind of canned cat food that is mostly fish bones and "by-products."

There are many different foods available, in such flavors as kidney, beef, liver and egg—all relished by baby raccoons. Always offer strictly fresh food. Give small bits at first, refrigerating the remainder.

OPOSSUM

Baby opossums will first begin taking bits of solid food at about two-and-a-half months of age. Such things as hard-boiled egg yolk, mashed banana, blended vegetables, and canned dog food are all good starter foods. Watch your fingers when letting baby opossums lick food. They have a mouth full of tiny needle-sharp teeth, which they quickly learn to use!

FEEDING SCHEDULE: BIRTH THROUGH WEANING

Raccoon					
	Birth to 2 weeks	2 to 4 weeks	4 to 6 weeks	6 to 8 weeks	8 weeks on
Milk	x	x	x	x	...
Hi-protein dry cereal	...	x	x	...	...
Cat food (small tins)	...	...	x	x	x
Puppy formula dry dog food	...	...	...	x	x
Feedings per day	12	12	8	4	3
Opossum					
Milk	x	x	x	x	...
Hi-protein dry cereal	...	x	x	x	x
Blended vegetables	...	...	x	x	...
Dog food	...	...	...	x	x
Vegetables or fruit	...	...	...	x	x
Feedings per day	24	20	12	10	5

Soon after the babies learn to eat solid foods, they will reject their bottle for good.

SYMPTOMS OF TROUBLE— AND WHAT TO DO

DIARRHEA

Diarrhea can be quite a problem in baby raccoons and opossums. The babies are so little that even mild diarrhea quickly kills them. If watched for closely, the diarrhea can be noticed at feeding time. Once the baby becomes dehydrated and begins acting depressed, chances of saving it are small.

As soon as diarrhea is noticed, stop all feedings of milk immediately. Milk is irritating to the intestinal tract and will only encourage the diarrhea to continue. Instead of the milk, give the baby an oral electrolyte solution, available at drugstores and from your veterinarian. When diarrhea is present, it dehydrates the body. In this process, not only are fluids lost, but also body salts and chemicals. These must be replaced, in addition to fluids, or the animal cannot live.

Give the electrolyte solution every two hours in place of normal feedings, and give kaolin-pectin, with neomycin added, every other hour.

You can give the babies about 5 cc of kaolin-pectin until they weigh 12 ounces or more; then give them 7 cc. You can measure it with a disposable syringe, minus the needle. Of course, very tiny opossum babies would take less. Use your own judgment.

Be sure to stimulate the babies after the electrolyte feedings. As soon as the diarrhea stops, you can discontinue the kaolin-pectin and electrolytes. When you begin feeding milk again, start with a half milk/half warm water solution for the first feeding.

CONSTIPATION

Constipation is usually only seen in these babies while their eyes are still closed. It can be caused by forgetting to stimulate elimination after a feeding. Often the baby will be found comatose or dead. If one is found looking full before a feeding and is acting weak, suspect constipation and give an enema with warm soapy water immediately. Don't wait "to see if it gets better." It will not.

Use your imagination for an enema syringe. A device that has worked for us is a feeding tube! The amount of the enema solution should be half the amount of the milk you feed the baby.

After results are obtained, recovery is usually uneventful, provided that the treatment has been given in time and the baby has not absorbed too much toxic material.

CHILL

On occasion, you may find a baby that has crawled away from the nest and has become chilled or the power supplying the heat source may have gone out, leaving all the babies chilled. They may appear dead at first, but immersing them in very warm (not hot) water for a few minutes generally brings about quick revival (of course, do not immerse the head!).

As soon as they begin to move about, dry them off, and place them in a warm box. Give them one feeding of Karo syrup and water, warmed to just above body temperature.

VACCINATIONS

It is recommended that baby raccoons be vaccinated against both canine and feline distemper, as they are susceptible to both. This vaccination is done at about six to eight weeks of age.

If the raccoon or opossum is kept past six months of age, it is a good idea to have it vaccinated with an inactivated rabies vaccine. This vaccination must be repeated annually.

GENERAL CARE

Both baby raccoons and opossums need a strong cage for the time between babyhood and release. Baby raccoons need the cage to protect them from their own mischief, and baby opossums need it to save them from their stupidity. (Very few animals are stupid, but opossums have a low mentality in the home.) If opossums are just left to run in the house, they are likely to hide behind the refrigerator, never coming out to eat. Or they will get lost in the living room, unable to find the way back into the kitchen where they are fed. Sometimes it seems as though they just forget to eat!

Baby raccoons, on the other hand, are bright and energetic. We had two eight-week-old babies flip the hook on their "bedroom" and escape, having the run of the house overnight. They loved the kitchen. There was peanut butter all over, mixed with jelly, honey, and broken eggs—along with the entire contents of the refrigerator and just about every pot and pan in the cupboard! The two babies sat with seemingly smug looks on top of the stove, handling the clock with very sticky paws.

Raccoons don't improve with age in this respect. We found that a 30-pound raccoon can make 10 times as much mess as a 3-pound one can! Raccoons are very curious and seem to have to handle everything they inspect—even peoples' eyeballs!

Both raccoons and opossums are very cute babies, but do not really adapt to captivity. As they grow older, both become aggressive, not because they have nasty temperaments, but from the loss of respect for human beings and from being pampered as babies. When they want to be left alone, they will bite if you try to touch them. When you are near their food, they bite. When they want down and you are holding them, they bite. And so forth.

When baby raccoons can be raised in comparative freedom, uncaged, and not treated like dogs or cats, they can grow up to be nice friends, but never pets.

SAFE RELEASE TO THE WILD

Both young raccoons and the young opossums are quite easily released into the wild. The key to a safe release lies in choosing the right territory. It should be fairly remote, as young animals that are raised in captivity often get into trouble by approaching strangers who do not have friendly intentions toward animals.

We usually take the babies into "their" area, along with a small bag of dry dog food. The food is placed in a spot that is sheltered from the weather, and the babies are introduced to the area. They usually snack a bit on the food, then wander off into the brush, never to return.

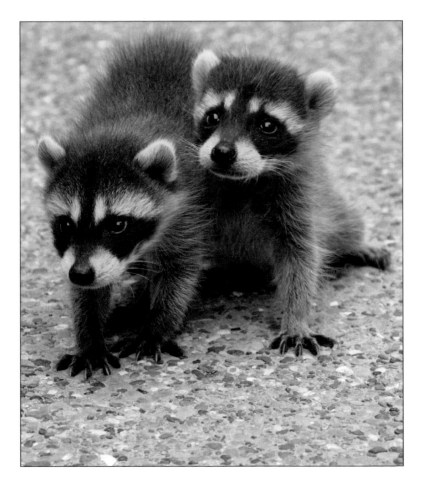

Bear Cubs

THERE IS NO "cuter" animal than a baby bear. There is also no more dangerous North American animal than a bear full grown. Even the smallest species of North American bear, the black bear, can kill a cow. Therefore, if you should come across a cute little baby bear cub "lost" in the woods, conjure up a vision of a huge, powerful, very aroused mother bear charging out of the brush to "rescue" her baby from you. In other words, be very sure that the cub you've found is an orphan!

Bear cubs are born while the female is in hibernation. They are very small, nearly naked, and look more like piglets than bears. Black bear cubs only weigh from 6 to 10 ounces at birth. There may be from one to four cubs in a litter, and twins are common. At two months of

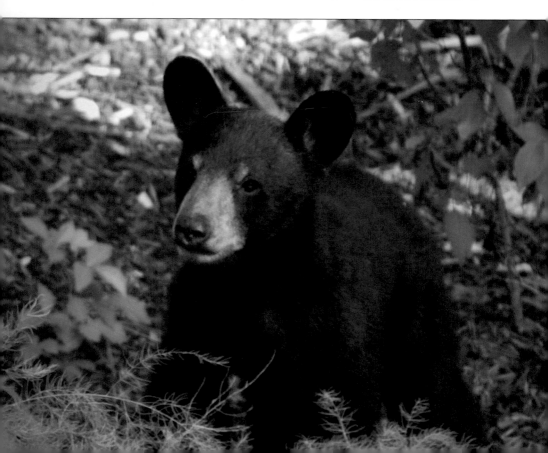

age, the cubs are still in the den with the mother. They have their eyes open, have a good coat of hair, but they are still unable to walk.

In the spring, often in late March and early April, the female emerges from the den with her cubs, now weighing from 5 to 7 pounds (black bear), from 10 to 15 pounds (grizzly). By late summer, the cubs can get along without their mother, but they are usually with her until their second spring.

Other than man, the infant bear's worst enemy is the adult male of the species. Male bears have nothing to do with raising the young. In fact, they regard cubs as a tasty snack. The female will do everything in her power to protect her cubs from hungry males and from any other threat, but on occasion, she is mortally wounded in the struggle. Sometimes a female bear is killed on the highway, often accompanied by her cubs.

If you find a bear cub that is genuinely in need of human assistance to survive, pack it up safely in a strong box for the trip home. Remember that a big, late summer cub, weighing 30 pounds or more will have a good chance of surviving in the wild and would best be left in the wild.

GAME REGULATIONS

It is necessary to contact your local game warden when planning to raise a bear cub. In most states, they are protected, and you risk a large fine by keeping one without permission.

THE INJURED CUB

Like their mothers, cubs are most often injured or killed by male bears and cars. An injured cub should be examined and treated by a veterinarian before being brought home. Do not try to set a broken leg yourself, as the bones are quite large and are difficult to get into alignment without using special equipment.

Do be careful in handling an injured cub, both to protect it from further injuries, and to protect yourself from bites and scratches. The best way is to shoo it into a strong box or drum and transport it in that same container.

Call the game warden for the phone number of your local wildlife rehabilitation center.

RAISING THE CUB

In general, you can raise the cub just as you would a human infant. Instead of a crib, though, the cub is best kept in a cage with a sturdy box for a bed. If the cub weighs less than 15 pounds, it should be kept in quite warm, draft-free quarters. A dog crate situated in the kitchen or bedroom works fine.

Remember, these small cubs rely on the heat of their mother's body for warmth when they are chilled. Without a mother to provide the extra heat, you will have to do it. A heating pad under one corner of the crate, or even a special armored heating pad made for puppies or baby pigs, may be necessary. A chilled cub is prone to sickness.

Although it may be tempting, do not allow the cub the unsupervised run of the house. Cubs climb a lot and get into about as much trouble as baby raccoons do!

The cub can be fed from either a human baby bottle or a pop bottle fitted with a lamb nipple. If fed every two hours (at two months) or every four hours (at two to four months), the cub can be allowed to have as much from the bottle as it will drink without encouragement. When the cub turns away from the nipple, don't coax it to have "just a little more." If this is done, the cub will soon develop indigestion and diarrhea.

The formula can either be goat milk, with children's liquid vitamins added, or a human baby formula, such as Enfamil with iron added.

After the cub is two months old, you can add high-protein baby cereal to the milk, feeding it from the bottle.

It is helpful to burp the cubs. In the wild, they nurse and then tumble about, following the mother. But, in captivity, cubs often curl up in a corner to sleep and get colicky pains and indigestion from not getting rid of air and gas.

Offer the cub small amounts of thickened cereal and milk, with canned dog food or hard-boiled egg yolk added every few days. Even quite young cubs soon learn to nibble solid foods. Mashed banana and other fruits are also relished early. A cub will suck on stale bread soaked in milk like a pacifier, and this makes an easy introduction to solid food, even while the cub is on the bottle for the bulk of the diet.

FORCE-FEEDING, WHEN NECESSARY

Some cubs come to us so weak from lack of food, or so depressed from injuries, that they refuse to suck from a bottle. In this case, the cubs must be force-fed, until they have regained their appetites. This can easiest be done with a stomach tube. (See the chapter *Pups.*) Give them four to eight ounces, depending on their size, every two hours, until they are more active and show interest in eating on their own.

When cubs are extremely weak, it is better to give them Karo syrup and warm water, mixed half and half, instead of milk. This will give them quick strength and energy, enabling them to become more active and be more able to absorb milk given at later feedings.

SYMPTOMS OF TROUBLE— AND WHAT TO DO

DEHYDRATION

Bear cubs are not so frequently bothered by diarrhea as are many other baby animals, and so they are not as bothered by dehydration because of it. But, newly found bear cubs do frequently suffer from dehydration if they are quite young and have been without a mother for some time. They don't drink much water at this age and can soon dehydrate. This can be discovered by grabbing the cub's skin and tugging it a little. It should be soft, pliable, and rubbery. If it feels tight and hard, the cub is probably dehydrated.

When a cub suffers from dehydration, it is necessary to give the cub an electrolyte solution before feeding it milk. When a cub dehydrates, it is deficient not just in body liquid, but in the normal body salts and chemicals necessary for life as well. And, when correcting dehydration, not only is it necessary to replace the fluid, but these lost salts and chemicals must also be replaced. If the cub shows an interest in sucking, it can be given one or two feedings of an oral electrolyte solution, available in the infant section of your drugstore, or from your veterinarian.

If the cub seems dejected and you believe it is dehydrated, your veterinarian should examine the cub. It may need injectable electrolytes, or possibly antibiotics or other medicines to fight diarrhea or an infection which has caused the dehydration.

INDIGESTION

As bear cubs get a little older, they begin to eat a wider variety of things. And they aren't too picky about what they do eat. Like a house dog, they can and will eat chicken bones, tinfoil, and highly spiced foods, if available (stolen from a table or from the trash, if necessary!), often to the discomfort of their digestive tracts.

The first signs of indigestion may be depression. A cub may not eat at mealtime. Then there may be colic. With a complete blockage, there will not be diarrhea. However, in most cases of indigestion the cub will soon have diarrhea.

If the cub is caught soon after having eaten a poor "food," it can be given a human dose of mineral or castor oil, both to aid in passing the material on through the digestive tract, and to coat the intestines so that it is not absorbed.

Following the oil dose by an hour, you can give a human dosage of Pepto-Bismol. This is generally enough to bring about quick relief. If not, see your veterinarian at once.

GENERAL CARE

Few people can live like bears, and bears certainly cannot live like people. Therefore, the bear cub, no matter how cute and affectionate, cannot be a year-round house pet. Both you and the bear will suffer. Bear cubs are constantly on the move, digging, exploring, and chewing. It is their nature. But, in a house, it is hard on the furniture, cupboards, and rugs.

We suppose we should mention zoos and parks, which are the fate of many cubs. True, you can visit the cub there and know his fate, but often these bears are not happy and live short, miserable lives. We are not talking, of course, about big, well-run zoos and animal parks, but we mean little local zoos, often tightly budgeted, or local "roadside zoos," which are often run with only profit—not the well-being of the animals—in mind.

In the wild, bear cubs remain with their mother for a year, learning to forage and hunt for themselves. A cub released in the fall will seldom survive on its own and should be kept over winter and released later on in the early summer after hibernation.

If the cub is to be wintered over, a sturdy cage for it is a must. The cage should be large (at least 20 by 20 feet), dry, and strong, constructed of heavy-gauge chain link. There should either be a concrete bottom to the pen, or the chain link should be buried at least 2 feet in the ground, with a good load of crushed rock dumped in the pen for drainage. The cage should be built next to a decent-size shed, so the bear cub can have a "den" out of the weather. The den should have a guillotine door, which can be raised and lowered from outside the pen. Many bear cubs stay docile through their first year, but some do get a bit rough, and cleaning the pen is much easier without a well-intentioned cub dragging on your leg! It's much easier to shut the cub in the den while cleaning up.

As fall approaches, increase the food. By now, the cub will be eating dry dog food, stale bread, slaughterhouse by-products, and fruit rejects from the market. Give the cub a good big pile of straw in the corner of the den to build a "nest" for hibernation, should the cub desire it. A few cubs don't really hibernate, but spend long periods in the nest, coming out to feed briefly from time to time. Be sure dry, fresh food is available should the cub emerge from the den. If the cub stays out for longer than a few minutes, offer water. Few bears eat or drink much after denning up, though, as the body does not excrete waste while the bear is in hibernation, and therefore, the bear usually does not have hunger or thirst after the deep rest begins.

Always keep in mind that your cub is growing quite large now and could harm a person, even if only accidentally. Do not let children—or any outside adults, for that matter—play with the cub. You might be willing to gamble on being bitten or cuffed, but if your cub were to injure someone else, you might be liable for a lawsuit—and the cub might be shot for a "killer" bear! People tend to be a little irrational when they are bleeding!

SAFE RELEASE TO THE WILD

When the cub is ready for release, you will generally know it. Instead of acting like a "little teddy bear," the cub begins acting more like an adult. It guards its food more emphatically, becomes more serious in searching for food outside the pen, and seems less dependent on you.

Perhaps the most important thing in releasing the cub to the wild is your choice of a site for the release. This should be a remote area, well away from other people, farms, and tourists. Many hand-raised cubs meet sad ends by being too friendly with nervous people or helping themselves to eggs, poultry, or other farm produce. The "cub" may be three years old and still act friendly, having little fear of humans. To a strange person, however, the "cub" may look awesome—especially if it is trying to get into the house, or if it wanders up onto the front lawn!

When possible, there should be no people within a 10-mile radius of the release site. The area should not be the territory of other wild bears, so look well for bear signs (such as claw marks on trees, tracks, and dead logs turned over in a search for grubs), before releasing the cub. Cubs are often attacked and killed by older male bears.

The area should also be rich in natural foods. Look for berry bushes and marshy areas, where tender grasses and frogs abound. Bears do not generally range in old, heavy woods, with little brush and grass present, as there is little food available there. Bears like tender grass, small rodents, insect larvae, acorns, wild fruits and berries, and insects.

If at all possible, try to camp in the vicinity for a few days so that the cub, now having its freedom, can explore the area, with you still around as moral support. Generally, the cub will explore further each day, finally choosing not to return to your camp. It would be a good idea to leave some dry dog food in a sheltered spot at the old campsite for the cub to call back on, should its first foraging trips be unsuccessful.

Medium-Size Rodents

SQUIRRELS, CHIPMUNKS, GOPHERS, WOODCHUCKS, and RABBITS

Squirrels (Grey, Red, Flying)

BABY SQUIRRELS ARE often tossed out of the nest, if not killed, by the male of the species. They are quite easily hand-raised and are very cute "temporary pets."

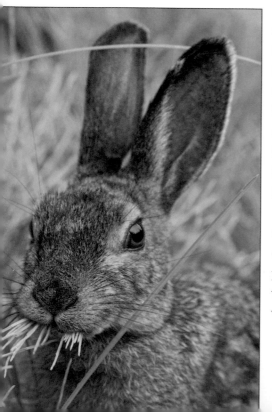

When baby squirrels are found, first check them for injuries. Broken legs and bites are common. Should a leg be broken, it would be best to take the squirrel to your veterinarian to have it set. If, however, you cannot afford this expense, you can try to set it yourself, following the directions in the chapter *First Aid and Follow-Up Care of Wounds*.

It's best to check your game regulations (call your game warden); in most states it's not legal to possess wild rodents and the game warden will often refer you to a local wildlife rehabilitation center to help raise the orphans you have found. Also, keep in mind the possibility of rabies in wildlife in your area; some states have a fairly common occurrence of rabies in wildlife. It's best to check with your veterinarian, and be sure to avoid bites at all cost.

Baby squirrels generally nurse quite readily on a doll bottle or a pet nurser, available at any pet shop. Be sure the bottle does have a soft rubber nipple, however.

The babies are born hairless, blind, and quite helpless. By three-and-a-half weeks to five weeks (flying squirrel, three-and-a-half weeks; red, four weeks; grey, five weeks), the babies' eyes are open, and they are furred out.

Squirrels at a very young age, still naked and blind, can be difficult to save, due to the small and very frequent feedings that are necessary. But once the squirrels are furred out well, they are usually quite easy to raise.

FEEDING

The baby squirrels should be fed a highly digestible formula, such as the human baby formula Enfamil (without iron) or goat milk. (Don't add Karo syrup or vitamins, or you may give them diarrhea.) This, fed from a bottle, should be given at least every two hours. Give the babies just enough to fill them up, but not so much that they are overfed.

As soon as the squirrels are well furred and the eyes open, you can begin adding a little high-protein dry baby cereal to the milk, keeping it thin enough to pass through the hole in the nipple.

Soon, they can nibble small amounts of cereal with milk out of a spoon.

Remember, when feeding very young squirrels, to stimulate them to urinate and pass solid wastes. This is done by massaging the abdomen and rectal area with a warm, damp cloth. Do this after each feeding until the babies are eliminating on their own. It is necessary to help them in this way, as they may become constipated or withhold their urine, becoming toxic.

Baby squirrels quickly learn to nibble on solid foods. Ours loved peanut butter on crackers, bread crusts, apples, bananas, unsalted peanuts, and sunflower seeds.

Do be careful in handling baby squirrels, as they have very sharp teeth and will nip if you frighten them.

SAFE RELEASE

Baby squirrels are quite easy to release. They will quickly become self-sufficient and learn to adapt to wild life with little problem, even in a city.

FEEDING SCHEDULE: BIRTH TO RELEASE

	Birth to 4 weeks	4 to 6 weeks	6 to 8 weeks	8 weeks on
Milk	x	x	x	...
Cereal	...	x	x	...
Bread	...	...	x	x
Fruits	...	...	x	x
Sunflower seeds	...	...	...	x
Feedings per day	12	9	6	free choice

At first, they will return for feed and human companionship, but soon they come back only for food from time to time—then hardly ever, since they are entirely happy with other wild squirrels.

Chipmunks, Gophers, Woodchucks, and Rabbits

Although many people would rather *not* raise these "sometimes pests," few people can resist those cute babies, which desperately need their help in order to survive.

FEEDING

As with baby squirrels, these babies must be fed small amounts, at least every two hours. They may be fed all they will readily take from a doll bottle with rubber nipple, or a pet nurser bottle, available at most pet shops. We generally use whole goat milk, with no additives. Vitamin drops, iron drops, or Karo syrup seem to cause diarrhea in these babies.

As soon as the eyes are open, you can add high-protein dry cereal to the milk, keeping it just thin enough to pass through the nipple.

At the same time, you can begin offering small amounts of solid food. The best time to do this is before a feeding when the babies are quite hungry.

Recommended first foods include mixed cereal and milk, bread soaked in milk, raw vegetable bits, crackers, and apple pieces.

FEEDING SCHEDULE: BIRTH TO RELEASE

	Birth to 2 weeks	2 to 4 weeks	4 to 6 weeks	6 weeks on
Milk	x	x	x	...
Cereal	...	x	x	x
Bread	...	...	x	x
Fruits	...	...	x	x
Sunflower seeds, nuts	...	...	x	x
Feedings per day	12	12	8	continual free fed

SAFE RELEASE

These babies are also quite easy to release. When they are eating on their own, whether in nature or when raised by humans, they are able to take care of themselves.

The main thing is to find a place to release them where there are no human enemies. The *worst* place to release them is near a farm or garden. These are places where small rodents are most disliked.

SYMPTOMS OF TROUBLE IN ALL MEDIUM-SIZE RODENTS— AND WHAT TO DO

DIARRHEA

There are several things that cause diarrhea in young rodents. Most common is overfeeding. Treatment for this is simply cutting down on the amount of milk fed at a few feedings.

Coccidiosis is a common cause of diarrhea in confined babies. It is caused by a one-celled internal parasite. Diarrhea is the most obvious symptom. It can easily be diagnosed by your veterinarian, by examination of a little sample of feces under a microscope. The cure is sulfamethazine which may be added to the drinking water or given by eyedropper.

Mucoid enteritis is also often seen in baby rodents, especially rabbits. It generally hits them at around three weeks of age, but can strike sooner or later. The stool usually contains a certain amount of mucus, and the baby feels "squishy" in the abdominal region. Emtryl is used to treat this condition and is given either in the water or by eyedropper. The label suggests proper dosage.

Dehydration occurs in all cases of diarrhea, no matter what the cause, and is usually what kills the babies. In dehydration, not only body fluid is lost, but also necessary body salts and chemicals. So, to help correct the condition, not only must fluid be given, but also these salts and chemicals, called electrolytes.

When treating diarrhea, it is very important to discontinue all milk being fed (it irritates the digestive tract and prolongs the diarrhea), and replace it with the same amount of an electrolyte solution, which can be bought at any drugstore, in the infant department.

	Blind, hairless baby	Baby with hair, eyes closed	Unweaned baby
Squirrel	2 cc	4 cc	5 cc
Flying squirrel	1 cc.	2 cc	3 cc
Chipmunk, Ground squirrel	1 cc.	2 cc	3 cc
Woodchuck	4 cc	6 cc	8 cc
Rabbit	2 cc	4 cc	5 cc

No matter what the cause of the diarrhea, it is often necessary to give a special medicine to stop the loose bowels, even when a drug is used to treat the *cause* of the diarrhea. A few drops of kaolin-pectin every two hours will usually help to halt common diarrhea. Use the table to assist you in determining the correct amount.

GENERAL CARE FOR ALL MEDIUM-SIZE RODENTS

When these babies are first brought into the home, it is very important to keep them warm. This is best done by placing them in a small box, warmed by a 100-watt light bulb. Place a thermometer inside the box after it has warmed up for 15 minutes. It should not be over 90°F, nor under 75°F.

If the babies are hairless, they will need a nest made of cotton, or some other soft, absorbent nesting material. As they grow and hair out, you can discontinue the use of the light bulb.

As soon as they are nibbling on solid food, they will also be moving about more, exploring their nearby surroundings. At this time, you should move them to a cage to prevent them from getting into trouble. (A tiny squirrel might be able to climb out of the nest, but would get lost on the floor.) The cage should be big enough to hold the babies up to the point that they are ready to release. The ideal cage has plenty of room for the babies to play around outside the nest. All babies that climb should be provided with a sturdy branch. Woodchucks and ground squirrels enjoy a pile of sand to roll and dig in.

It is a good idea to dust all rodent babies for fleas with a good, safe rotenone powder, as they are quite prone to fleas and lice, often picked up from the mother shortly after birth.

Water can be supplied from a drinking bottle to prevent a damp cage caused by playful spills.

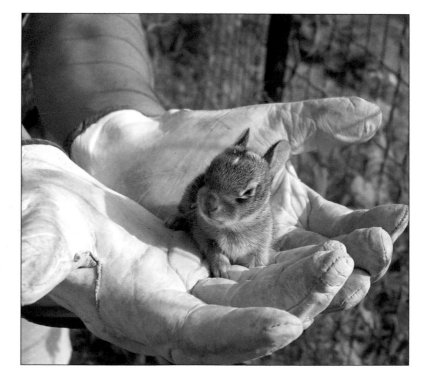

Small Rodents

MICE, HAMSTERS, GERBILS, and RATS

HERE, WE GET into the "least cute" of all baby animals, the ones few people bother with—and the babies "least likely to succeed." Should you be presented with a bunch of bean-size, pink, blind, and hairless babies to raise, be prepared to fail. In nature, the mother feeds the litter very often, more often than you will be able to. However, once the babies start to have a fur covering, your chances improve considerably. There are a few special problems with these little babies that are

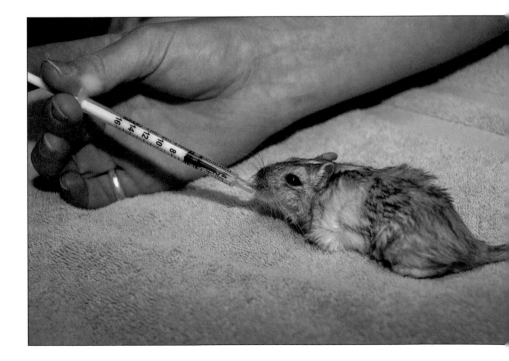

not encountered in raising other babies. The biggest one is the size of the mouth—much too small to suck from even a tiny doll bottle. We have found that a piece of absorbent string, acting like a wick from bottle to baby, works as well as anything, until the babies are large enough to grasp the nipple itself.

Remember that these babies only weigh a fraction of an ounce, so they are very easily injured by even gentle handling.

And, remember that they only need a very few drops of milk at a time. Do not overfeed.

Otherwise, their care is identical to that of the larger rodents, discussed in the previous chapter.

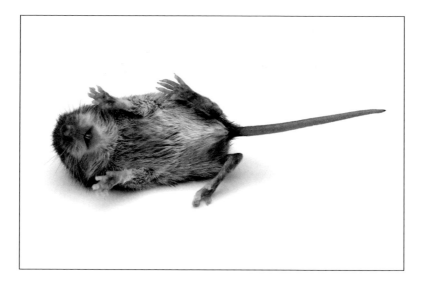

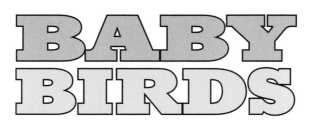

Raptors

OWLS, HAWKS, and EAGLES
NESTING HABITS

THE BIRDS OF prey build very loose nests. The best consist of a big pile of sticks and branches, packed together to form a nesting place. The nests are usually quite high up, resting in the tops of trees, on rocky ledges, and in hollow trees (owls). Burrowing owls nest in the ground, often in abandoned prairie dog holes. From one to five eggs are laid, and from the time those eggs hatch, it is very easy to distinguish the chicks as birds of prey. Their grasping talons are very large, and their hooked beaks, meant for grasping prey, are prominent.

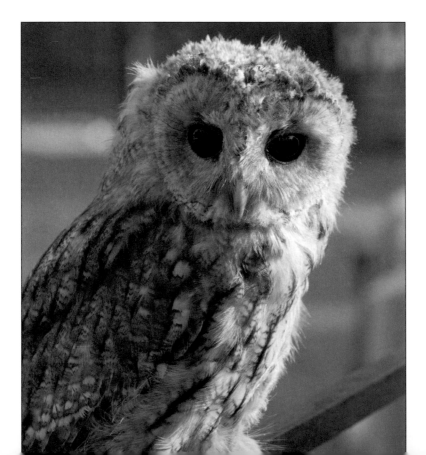

FINDING CHICKS

Now and then, a person may find a small, flightless owl or hawk chick on the ground. Whenever possible, try to locate the nest and replace the fallen chick. One word of caution, though: be careful when doing this, as the irate parents will not know you are trying to help and may attack you as you climb about holding the squalling chick.

If the nest is far up a hard-to-climb tree or rocky cliff, it is generally best to take the chick to a wildlife rehabilitation center, rather than risk your life by climbing up to the nest. Even an experienced falconer has been known to let loose of a branch and fall when attacked by a large hawk.

All birds of prey are protected, and it is illegal to possess one without being licensed and having permits to do so. Disregarding these laws, no matter how good your intensions are, makes you liable for hefty fines and possible imprisonment! When finding an orphaned raptor chick, call your game warden to find out the phone number of the nearest wildlife rehabilitation center immediately.

If you are licensed and permitted to raise raptor chicks, the following information may help.

IDENTIFYING THE CHICK

Identification of the chick is important. Without knowing the species, you will not know for sure what the natural foods are. And, to have the best chance of rearing the chick, you must come close to the natural foods in feeding them. For instance, a sparrow hawk eats many insects, and few small rodents and frogs, and an eagle eats very few insects. Some of these birds eat mainly fish. It is up to you to find this out. If the parents are present, make mental notes as to their color and size. Later, you can match up this description with a picture in a good bird book.

When the parents are not available, you have a harder time identifying the chicks, as they do not have their adult color for several weeks after leaving the nest. If there is an ornithologist or a naturalist nearby, take the chick in for identification. Otherwise, you might contact your game warden. You should do this anyway, as all birds of prey are protected by law, and you must be permitted by law to raise the chick.

If you can find no one to help identify the chick, you will have to first feed it (small pieces of liver usually are a good first food, regardless of the species), then go to the library and search through bird books, until you can identify "your" chick. As you do this, keep in mind common birds of prey in your area and check them first.

DETERMINING THE AGE OF THE CHICK

It is also important to get a pretty good idea of how old the chick is, in order to give it correctly timed feedings. Most predatory chicks remain in the nest, unable to fly for 5 to 12 weeks, depending on the adult size.

Soon after hatching, they are all legs, talons, and beak, and are covered with a light fluff. All chicks in the nest do not hatch at once, so there are often chicks ranging from newly hatched to beginning to feather out in the same clutch.

The chicks do not generally leave the nest until they are able to fly and are quite

FEEDING

When the chick is first brought home, it may refuse to take offered meat bits. When this happens, force-feeding is necessary. You can place a small piece of meat on a pencil (the eraser end), and tap at the back corner of the mouth. When the chick opens up, gently poke the meat way in and withdraw the pencil. Generally only one or two feedings of this sort are needed.

If the chick is very stubborn, you may have to pry the beak open *carefully*, from the back corner, with your fingernail. But remember, even a baby chick has a razor sharp beak and moves as fast as lightning at times. As soon as the chick begins to open its mouth, get the meat right there to be eaten—and protect your finger.

Very young chicks are best fed small amounts every three hours, day and night. As they begin to feather out, let them have all they will take every four hours, day and night. Predatory birds feed their chicks whole foods, including skin, hair, bone, and intestinal contents. Keep this in mind when hand-raising chicks. It may not be "nice," but those indigestible ingredients are necessary for the health of the chicks. Every few days, the chicks pass castings, which are hard balls of this indigestible material. It is necessary for proper digestion and bodily functions.

Very young chicks may be given bits of meat, rolled in bonemeal (available at your feed dealer) and a multiple liquid vitamin. As soon as the chicks are large enough, you can feed them whole, small mice. These mice can often be caught in traps in your attic or barn.

Never feed mice if you have rodent poison around. The mice may have taken some of the poisoned bait, and this poison could kill the chick.

Other feeds readily available are chicken necks, whole smelts, beef by-products, and a special food, Hills Carnivorous Bird Food, available at many pet shops and from veterinarians.

Remember, when choosing food for your chick, feed it as close to a natural diet as possible.

Don't make the mistake of feeding hamburger or stew meat, exclusive of any whole rodents, or other unappetizing foods. The chick will certainly die.

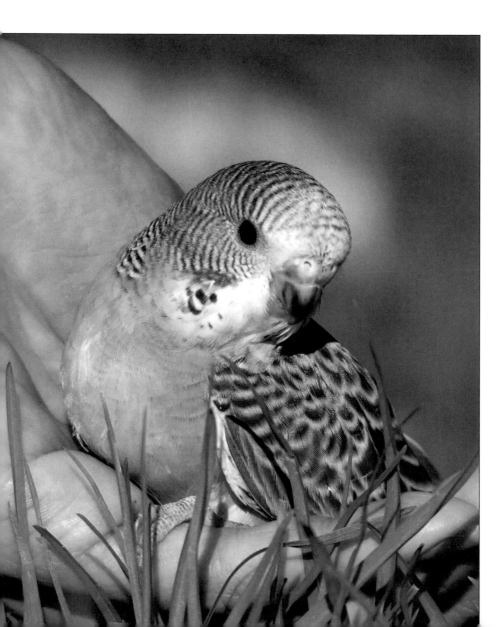

Song Birds

THE MOST COMMONLY hand-raised birds are song birds, including ordinary house birds such as the canary and parakeet. These small birds abound in woods, fields, and gardens. The parents often nest right in your backyard or under the eaves of the house. We will include here some birds that are not technically classed as "song birds"—sparrows and starlings, regarded by some people as pests. Many homes have canaries and parakeets for pets. Both kinds of birds breed fairly easily. They generally take very good care of their babies, but on occasion the young must be hand-raised.

FINDING BABY BIRDS

Most often, the baby birds that you find on the garden path or in the front yard have just fallen out of the nest. Baby birds are very "bottom heavy," and clumsy. Search thoroughly for the nest. Look in heavy brush, hollow tree branches, and in shrubbery close to the area where you found the baby. If you can find the nest, by all means deposit the baby back in the nest. Even if you find another nest of a similar bird with nestlings in it, put the baby there, rather than try to rear it yourself. This is especially true if the baby is naked and blind. Birds will not "smell" you on their babies.

We have had very good luck replacing babies—even in other nests. We have an old mother starling who nests in a hollow poplar tree in our front yard. She has raised two baby barn swallows three different years for us. We do wonder what she thinks when they begin to fly after insects though!

If the bird is feathered out, but cannot fly yet, look about you for nervous parents. If you do see scolding parents nearby, place the baby in some cover and leave it there. When the parents are watching the baby, they will also feed it and protect it to the best of their ability.

Should no parents or nests be available, the baby will need to be hand-raised.

WHAT KIND OF BABY IS IT?

When you find that baby, take it home and put it in a very warm place. A small, artificially heated box is best. Baby birds can not keep warm enough by themselves to sustain life when they are very small. A heating pad underneath a box, protected by an upside down cookie sheet helps a lot. Keep the heat on low or medium, not high. You want the temperature a few degrees lower than the birds' normal body temperature as possible, not hot enough to cause them distress. Generally, the smaller the species of bird, the higher the normal body temperature is. For instance, a sparrow and lark have a normal body temperature of about 112 degrees F, where a cardinal, starling, and pigeon have a normal temperature of about 110 degrees. Larger birds, such as a pheasant's or hawk's temperature is about 108 degrees, and an emu has a normal body temperature of about 102 degrees. Thus, a chicken with a normal body temperature of about 106 degrees would need about 99 degrees to comfortably warm a new chick. Or a sparrow, with a normal body temperature of 112 degrees, would need about 105 degrees to comfortably brood a baby.

If the young bird pants or has his mouth open, breathing, the heat is too warm; reduce it. If he is noisy and complains or is cool feeling and lethargic, he is too cold; increase the heat slightly. Then, before feeding it, try to figure out what kind of bird it is. Unless you know this, you will not be able to feed it correctly. You can't give a seed-eater bits of meat, nor an insect-eater seeds!

Study as many bird books as you can find. Hints you might use are the size of the baby, the area where it was found, and the birds commonly seen there. If the baby is beginning to feather out, you can get a good idea of the adult coloration. Look at the baby's beak. Birds that are strictly seed-eaters usually have quite a heavy beak as do the canary and parakeet, while insect-eaters have a longer beak that is not as thick.

When it really is impossible to tell for sure what kind of baby you have, you can feed it a mixture of stale bread, hard-boiled egg yolk, and well-mashed canned dog food. This will provide a little meat and vegetable, along with "seed," in the form of the wheat in the bread. It usually will suffice until the bird grows a little more, thereby enabling a positive identification.

DETERMINING THE AGE OF THE BABY

It is important to try to determine the approximate age of the baby, so you will know how warm it should be kept and how often it should

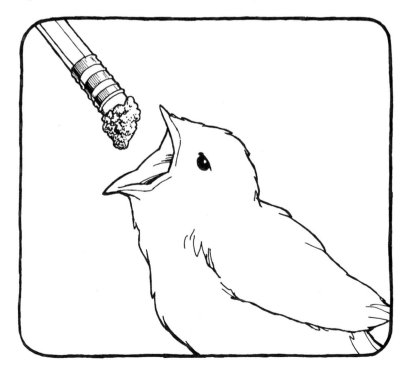

be fed. Most garden birds are in the nest for about five weeks. You can guess at the age by size and the amount of feathering the baby has.

FEEDING

Baby birds are very difficult to raise if they are not yet feathered out. The biggest reason for this is that they must be fed at least every half hour throughout the daytime. And, we do mean *every* half hour! If one feeding is skipped, the baby becomes severely weakened, often dying, regardless of care given after the skipped meal.

You may skip the midnight feedings, as the mother bird would be roosting, but get up at dawn to resume bird hours.

Meat-eaters (those that eat insects, worms, and beetles) can be fed bits of raw hamburger, good quality canned dog food, and natural foods gleaned from the garden or field. Be careful never to feed birds with insects taken from an area that has been sprayed or dusted with an insecticide.

Seed-eaters, such as canaries, parakeets, and finches, can be fed an unmedicated chick starter, mixed with a small amount of water, just enough to make the mixture crumbly, not dry, supplemented with mashed, hard-boiled egg yolk.

Some birds, such as starlings and sparrows, eat a wide variety of foods. These birds may have a variety of any of the above foods.

Baby birds are quite easy to feed in most instances, gaping their mouths open wide when hungry. Generally, all you have to do is make a small noise to make them aware you are there, and the mouths fly open with cheeps of anticipation. If a newly found baby will not open its mouth, try tapping the beak with a small stick which holds the morsel of food. A broom straw works well. If this still doesn't cause the baby to open its mouth, gently grasp the bird and pry open the beak from the back corner and insert the food particle.

Feed the baby all it will eat, within reason, at each feeding. Keep in mind how much the mother would bring each trip, and divide that by the usual number of young in the nest—often three or four.

Shore Birds

INCLUDED AMONG THE shore birds are all birds found at
the water's edge, such as gulls, rails, coots, herons, bitterns, terns, and
egrets. Because of the nesting habits of these birds (they lay their eggs
on land, not in trees), the nests are often raided by otters, raccoons,
opossums, and predatory birds. This may leave one or more babies
destitute, as they are often kicked out of the nest in the attack.

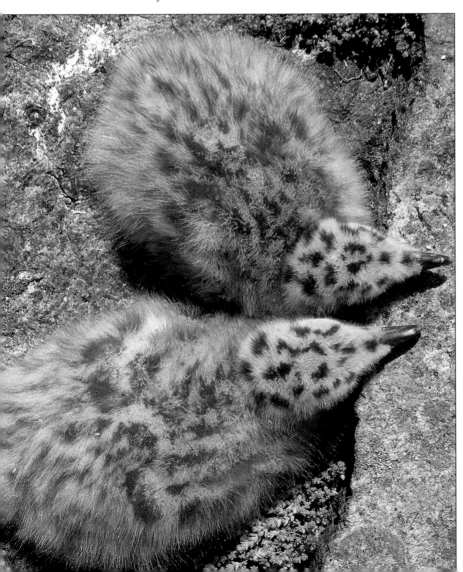

Other disasters such as nests washed out by high water, young birds somehow separated from the nest, and so on, result in baby shore birds that need human assistance to survive.

IDENTIFYING THE BABY BIRD

In order to feed the bird correctly, you will need to identify it. Some shore birds feed on worms and other insects, found in the mud. Others only eat fish.

If the baby does not have many feathers, you will have a harder time identifying it. Try to find a game warden, naturalist, or local person, familiar with shore birds, to help in the identification. If this does not work, study some good bird books at your local library for a clue to the correct identification.

Keep in mind the location where you found the bird, its size, and general build. Remember the adult size when trying to place the species of a baby. A baby great blue heron will be much larger than a baby bittern.

Remember that most shore birds are protected; contact your game warden for information on game laws. In many cases, it is unlawful to possess a wild shore bird, even if you intend on raising it to release. The warden may recommend that you take the bird to a nearby wildlife rehabilitation center that is licensed and permitted to raise wild shore bird babies.

DETERMINING THE AGE OF THE BABY

The newly hatched shore birds are nearly naked and weak. In a little over a week's time, they are feathered with a light fluff—except for coots and rails, whose babies wear fluff from the moment of hatching and are quite able to forage when first hatched.

As the babies get older, they also gain feathering, steadiness of legs, and body size. By six weeks of age, they are little miniatures of their adult counterparts, needing little assistance to get along.

FEEDING

We have had good success feeding finely chopped whole minnows to these babies. They must be fed every hour at the very least, every half hour if they are very small. It is a good idea to dip the minnow bits, at least once a day, in a powdered multivitamin. A good quality fish-based, canned cat food also works well. Do not feed a food that is very cheap and contains more fish bones and cereal than nutritious food.

The worm and insect-eaters of the marsh can be fed canned dog food, again of a good quality, and containing little cereal. A few drops of a liquid vitamin supplement should be added to the day's food, be well mixed, then kept refrigerated. Each feeding should be warmed up to body temperature for very young birds. For older juveniles, just warm refrigerated foods to room temperature.

Waterfowl

THE YOUNG OF waterfowl, tame or domestic, are among the easiest of all baby birds to hand-raise. And, for some reason, one finds few of these wild babies in need of human assistance. Perhaps the wild babies are so self-sufficient that either they live or they are eaten by predators; seldom are they orphaned or left in need.

Only a very young baby waterfowl needs human assistance to survive, unless it is injured.

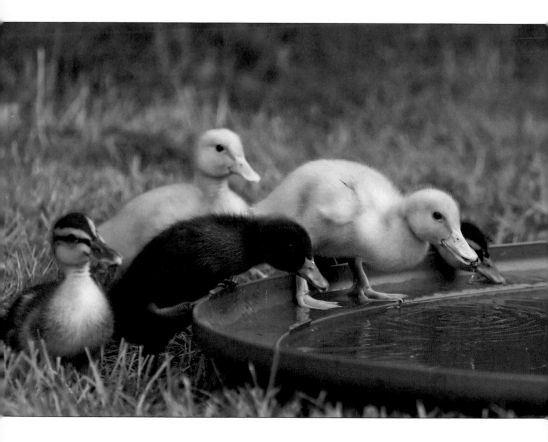

CARE AND FEEDING OF WATERFOWL BABIES

These babies are easiest started in a large cardboard box, with a heat lamp in one corner. They should be provided with heat until they replace down with feathers. A thick coat of newspapers should be placed on the bottom of the box, as they splash and spill water, making a big mess in a little time. They must not be allowed to stay damp for any length of time. For this reason, they should not be allowed to swim until they have feathered out. In the wild, they swim after the parents, but afterward, they climb out of the water on a bunch of dry grass and thoroughly dry out. In the box, they do not dry out and can soon take a chill and die.

Feeding is a simple matter. There is starting mash for ducks available at nearly every feed store. This should be provided free choice. *Never* water the babies *after* giving dry mash. They will drink, which pushes the dry mash into the digestive tract in a big mass, where it quickly forms an impaction or even chokes the bird.

Never give waterfowl babies chick starter or growing mash. This contains antibiotics, which will often kill young waterfowl. Keep all food given to waterfowl clean and fresh. Stale food is not unpalatable, but can contain harmful bacteria which quickly kills the unfortunate duck, goose, or whatever eats it.

FISHING BIRDS

There are some birds, which look like ducks or geese, but are really hunters of minnows. These are grebes, loons, cormorants, and the so-called fish ducks. They cannot be fed dry duck starter, as they are fish-eaters. When starting babies, use either a good-quality canned cat food with a fish base, or minnows that have been chopped finely. Use the entire fish, not just the fillet.

It is no time at all before the babies are feathered out and able to eat whole minnows and small smelts. When they have their entire coat of feathers, place them in a shallow pool of water and teach them to retrieve minnows from the water. Use dead minnows at first, then dying minnows, and finally fresh, sparkling, swimming fish. You can use the bathtub for this lesson, but we had a grebe that broke its neck diving into the bathtub after minnows. Since then, we have used either a stock tank or a child's plastic wading pool, as the sides give a bit when struck.

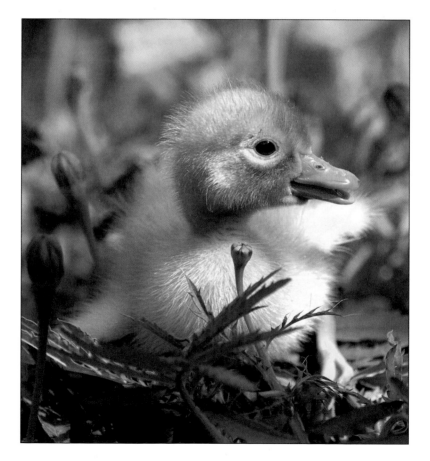

Domestic and Wild Poultry

CHICKENS, PHEASANTS, TURKEYS, and QUAILS

THE YOUNG OF these birds (for ease, we'll call them chicks, even though turkey babies are called poults) are also quite easy to raise.

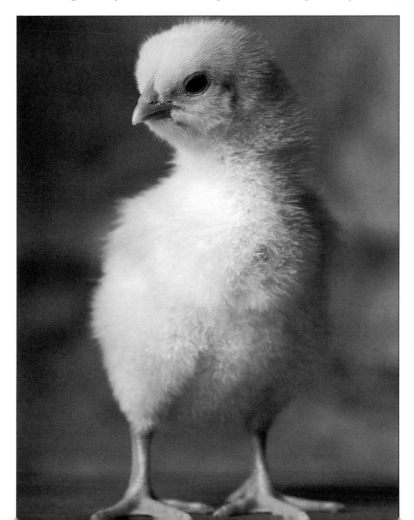

We have picked up several quail and pheasant chicks on the roadside, after their mother was struck and killed by a car. Running down the little balls of fluff can be quite a chore, especially when they reach the grass and hide, remaining perfectly motionless. It is hard to hunt, for fear of accidentally stepping on a hidden baby.

CARE AND FEEDING TIPS

These chicks can be housed either in a regular brooder or in a cardboard box with a heat lamp in one end. Wild chicks can be fed either a game bird starter, which is available at many feed stores, or a regular chick starter, which is available nearly everywhere feed is sold. If the chicks are very young, you may have to teach them how to eat. This is done by dropping small pieces of feed in front of them. The bits bounce on the floor and get the chicks' attention. Soon they will begin picking at the mash. When one chick begins to eat, the rest will soon follow.

Water for a few chicks can be supplied easiest in chick waterers, which hold an inverted jar of water and become self-filling. If tiny quail chicks are being raised, it is wise to sprinkle the trough area of the waterer with small pebbles, as the chicks can drown in an inch of water when they are very young.

They must be provided with heat until they have feathered out, such as a heat lamp hung securely above one end of the box. The temperature under the light should be 95 degrees for the first week of chick's life. Have enough room in the box for them to get away to a cooler spot if they choose.

Be sure to keep the box bedded with layers of dry newspaper, as dampness will soon cause chilling and death. Use the newspapers, instead of sawdust, as young chicks will pick at sawdust and eat it, which often causes an impaction and death.

General Information on All Birds

BE SURE THAT you are legally holding your baby bird. Many birds, especially migratory birds and birds of prey, are protected by law. And, there are stiff fines and legal harassment for people who keep them, even with the idea of release in mind.

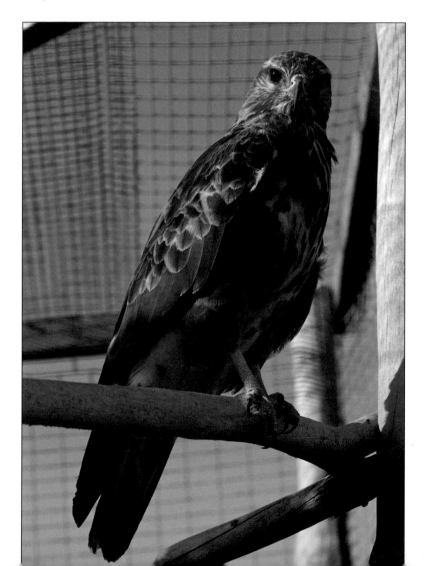

As soon as you bring any baby bird into the home, be sure you dust it well with rotenone powder, as almost all baby birds are infested with mites and/or lice. Rotenone is the safest insecticide available, and it will kill the vermin before they infest your house or seriously harm the baby bird. For the same reason, do not keep the baby's nest, if it is found with the baby. The nest will almost certainly be alive with "bugs."

Always be sure that the cage the growing bird is in is big enough for it. All large birds need room enough to stretch their wings as they are growing. This cannot be done in a cage so small that the bird can only sit on a branch all day. When in doubt, use a larger cage. No bird has ever suffered from too big a cage.

A flight cage is a good place to let the young bird test itself, without subjecting it to the dangers of the wild or those in your house. (Many birds are injured by hitting windows and household furnishings when learning to fly. They are also injured by trying to land on slippery surfaces, such as linoleum or counter tops.) The flight cage should be built so it is tall enough for you to work in standing up, and large enough to allow the bird you are raising to fly some distance, before having to land or turn around. At least one good-size tree branch should be provided for a perch. The bark should be left on. Clean sand can be sprinkled on the bottom of the cage weekly, with all dropping piles removed at the same time. The bird should be given food daily, and what is not eaten should be removed to prevent rodent infestation and to keep the food fresh, appetizing, and bacteria-free.

Fresh water should be provided for all birds. It should be deep enough for the bird to bathe in, but not so deep that it might fall in and drown. Even waterfowl should have stepping stones to get out of a pool.

Protection must be given against bad weather and the sun.

SECTION 4

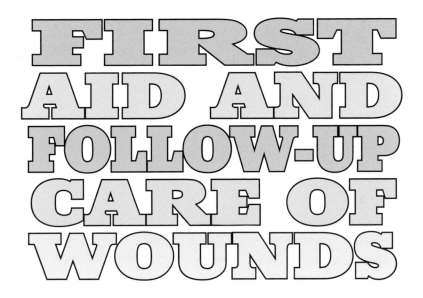

FIRST AID AND FOLLOW-UP CARE OF WOUNDS

This is *not* a chapter on being your own "do-it-yourself" veterinarian. Injuries are best treated by an experienced veterinarian with the correct instruments, sutures, drugs, and knowledge of anatomy that is needed for success. However, we do realize that many people cannot afford to take each and every small baby to their veterinarian for treatment of injuries. For instance, how many people are able, or willing, to spend even $15 to have a veterinarian set the broken leg on a baby sea gull?

We will attempt to show the best methods of home treatment and nursing afterward, and the dangers of a job incorrectly done.

Bite Wounds

MANY BABY ANIMALS are found suffering from bite wounds. This is not only because baby animals are the favored prey of dogs and cats, but often males of the same species. Some male animals, such as wolves, are very good parents—but others, such as squirrels, will kill their young at any opportunity.

There are many factors to consider in a bite wound, besides the punctures themselves.

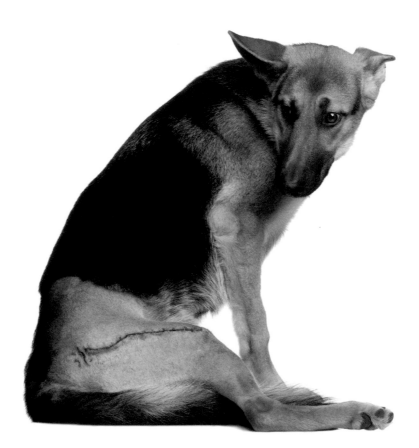

INTERNAL BLEEDING

Few bite wounds cause more than superficial external bleeding, unless extensive ripping has been done. In such a case, though, the baby seldom survives the attack. It is the crushing which occurs during the attack that causes internal injuries and hemorrhage, injuries much more dangerous to the animal than any external bite wounds generally are.

Suspect internal bleeding in all bite victims, and treat accordingly. Do not pick the baby up around the body, even with a towel or heavy gloves. This can aggravate the bleeding, possibly punching a broken rib through a lung. Instead, either push the baby into a box, carefully carrying it home, or pick the baby up by the loose skin at the back of the neck, close to the head to avoid being bitten. When the baby is carried by the skin, there will be no pressure at any point on the body. The skin will act as a sack, enclosing all the body with support. It is *not* advisable to carry healthy babies this way, as it is uncomfortable and can bruise the neck area.

If the baby is taken to a veterinarian, he can administer an injectable clotting drug which will stop all but severe bleeding.

Lacking this type of drug, you must keep the baby in a dark, warm box, completely away from all disturbing elements.

SHOCK

Shock is very common in bite injuries. There are several reasons: not only are the injuries painful, but also fright and internal injuries quickly induce shock. The animal in shock will appear depressed, quiet, and often cold. The mucous membranes in the eyelids and gums will appear very light colored, not a normal pink. Shock can be very serious, especially if not treated right away. It is often the number one killer of baby animals.

It is most important to get the animal into a warm, quiet place. You can put it in a cardboard box with a heating pad, first on high, then on low as it warms up to a normal body temperature. (See Appendix.) Take care, however, not to overheat the baby. This will cause the mucous membranes to redden and throw the baby into convulsions.

If possible, try to get a mixture of two parts warm water and one part Karo syrup into the baby with a feeding tube. Do not try to give it with a teaspoon or eyedropper, as you might cause the baby to inhale droplets into the lung.

TREATMENT OF THE WOUNDS THEMSELVES

Treatment consists of trimming away all hair or feathers in the near vicinity of the wound, as they will mat down over the wounds, trapping bacteria. This causes infection in a large number of cases. Do not worry about having them sewn up. Sutures are seldom needed in animal injuries. Only fresh wounds can be sutured, as older wounds are contaminated with bacteria and debris. When this material is closed in, infection rapidly sets in. When in doubt, contact your veterinarian.

Really, the only treatment needed is to keep the wounds cleaned out and soaked with a mild, but effective antiseptic.

It is also a good idea to keep the baby on a sulfa, such as sulfamethazine, or antibiotic until the wounds begin to heal—usually three to five days.

If possible, the animal should receive a tetanus antitoxin injection, as the tetanus organism loves warm, airless wounds.

CAUTION

Any animal that has received a bite wound should be treated with caution. Rabies is a very real problem, especially with wild animals. Rabies is a deadly virus, carried in the saliva of infected animals' mouths. Wild animals often found with rabies include skunks (the most common carrier), raccoons, foxes, and coyotes. Any warm-blooded animal can become infected with rabies through the infected saliva of an affected animal. It is not even necessary to actually be bitten. The saliva can be dripped into a scratch or common break in the skin such as a pimple or a hangnail.

The incubation period varies from two weeks to longer than a year. This means that an animal that has been in contact with a rabid animal can harbor the disease for longer than a year before showing symptoms. But once symptoms are noticed, the disease progresses rapidly, killing the animal within two weeks' time.

Symptoms vary with the two types of rabies—furious rabies and dumb rabies. Both are caused by the same organism, and both are deadly. Neither type responds to treatment, in humans or animals, once the symptoms are present.

Furious rabies is the most widely known. This is the "mad dog" variety. The affected animal exhibits odd behavior. A wild animal appears suddenly tame and unafraid. Animals that are timid become bold and aggressive. The animal may wander a long way from its natural territory. A young calf may suddenly act like an enraged bull, attacking much larger cattle. A skunk will often bite, instead of spraying. The affected animal may hallucinate, snapping at imaginary foes.

The animal affected by dumb rabies often becomes paralyzed in the throat and jaw. The mouth often hangs open, with saliva drooling uncontrollably from it. The animal cannot eat or drink. The voice may change. This form of rabies seldom produces animals that bite. They just sit in a corner, looking as though they swallowed a bone. Many times this is the reason people become infected. The person, thinking that the animal has swallowed a foreign object, reaches into the animal's mouth, comes in contact with the saliva which, in turn, infects a small scrape or cut, and the person begins incubating the disease, usually unknown to him.

This is not to say that all babies, or even many, that are found with bite wounds are carrying rabies. Far to the contrary. Rabies, fortunately, is quite uncommon. *But*, keep rabies in mind. Any baby animal that has been handled by you and then dies should be under suspicion if:

— it has exhibited any personality changes

— it has had any signs of throat paralysis

— it has bitten a person

— a person has had contact with the saliva (keep tube-feeding in mind)

If you are unsure about the conditions of such an animal's death, it would be best to have the head, or entire animal, sent into the state laboratory for examination.

Car Injuries

WE SEE MANY, many baby animals every year that have been struck by cars. Injuries range from fatal to barely stunned. Often, though, if the animal survives past 12 hours, the chances of an aided recovery are quite good.

CONCUSSION

Concussion is very common in automobile injuries. If the animal's head has not struck the car itself, it often receives a blow from a tire or muffler, or it strikes the hard-packed roadside.

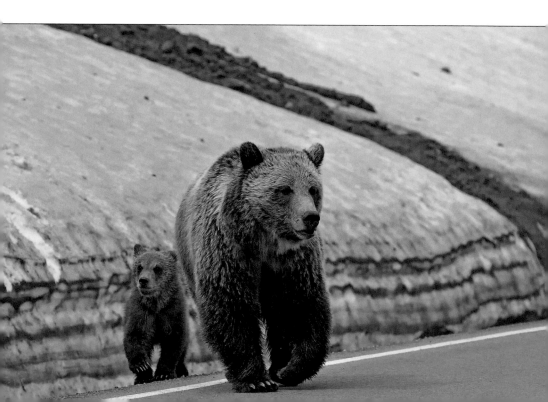

Concussions range from mild, with no visible signs, to severe, which are often fatal. In the majority of cases, the concussion is in the middle of this range. The animal may not be able to stand, falling to one side. Or it may be able to stand, but not balance, circling to one side. There is often dilation of one pupil, but not the other. The animal's head may be tipped to one side, and it might be unable to straighten up.

The best home treatment is a dark, draft-free, quiet box, well bedded so the animal cannot do itself further injury if it falls over. The baby may have to be tube-fed until it regains its balance. It is best to wear light plastic gloves for your protection (see rabies caution, page 161), as a rabid animal can act like one with a concussion.

BRUISES

Bruises are common, following an encounter with a car. They may swell somewhat, becoming hard lumps. Soon after the accident, cold packs may help stop the bleeding. (Remember that bruises are actually bleeding under the skin.) Unless they are very severe, they are seldom dangerous.

SCRAPES AND SCRATCHES

These injuries are also commonly seen. All hair or feathers should be trimmed away from the area. If they are not, they will stick to the injuries, causing rapid infection. With birds, the best thing to do is to pluck the feathers from the area, as they will grow back much sooner if plucked than if cut. A light antiseptic ointment can be applied daily, until healing is complete. Do not use a heavy salve as it only picks up dirt, hair, feathers, and bits of food, all of which retard healing and could cause an infection.

The use of a *light* ointment is necessary. As with floor-burn-type scrapes and scratches, the skin often thickens and hardens, and will slough off, unless kept soft and pliable.

GRAVEL PUNCTURE

Examine all animal babies found on the roadside for gravel which has punctured the skin. (If you have ever run on a cinder track, you know how gravel can travel way up under the skin on impact.) The gravel will appear quite close under the skin, like little dark bumps. It must be removed, or an abscess or infection will often follow.

When the gravel has not traveled too far from the point of entry, just have a helper restrain the animal, and pick out the pieces with a pair of long-nosed tweezers. But, if the gravel has worked way up under the skin, you may have to cut down on the bump with a razor blade to remove it. Sterilize the blade and work carefully. After the gravel has been removed, wash the area thoroughly with hydrogen peroxide.

It is a good idea to keep the animal on an antibiotic or sulfa for five days, following the removal of gravel as there will probably be small bits of dirt under the skin, and they might cause an infection.

EYE INJURIES

On occasion, the car itself does little damage, but as the animal or bird lands on the roadside, dirt or gravel is thrown into the eye. Such animals are often found wandering on the road itself, with great streams of tears flowing down the cheeks.

Be sure you do not get bitten while treating, and carefully rinse the eyes, one at a time, with warm, distilled water and boric acid. Try to rinse every tiny particle of sand and gravel from the eye. Be sure to lift each lid, to examine for pieces lodged there. As soon as the eye is perfectly clear, check for tiny punctures in the eyeball itself. If you can see none, the chances of complete recovery are good.

From the drugstore or your veterinarian try to get an ophthalmic (eye) ointment that contains both an antibiotic (or sulfa) and a local anaesthetic, such as tetracaine or procaine. The antibiotic will help prevent infection, and the local anaesthetic will soothe the pain. In severe cases, it is best to cover the affected eye, to prevent light from further irritating it.

SHOCK AND INTERNAL INJURIES

Both shock and internal injuries are also common in automobile accidents (see Index). It is best to restrain the suspected animal in a warm cardboard box for a day or two following the accident, as this is the best home treatment for both conditions.

Feed the suspected animal lightly for a day or two, as the animal with internal bleeding or shock cannot readily absorb foods, and large masses of food in the digestive system could aggravate either condition.

Broken Limbs and Other Serious Injuries

MAMMALS

MANY BABY ANIMALS are found with broken legs. As their legs are quite small, especially tiny babies, they are very prone to injuries. In many cases, the limb will dangle, uselessly, and there will often be swelling in the area of the trauma.

In many cases, broken legs are among the easiest of injuries to heal. This, of course, depends on proper care and treatment.

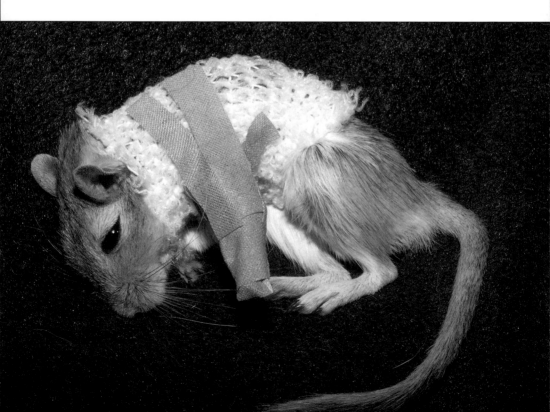

It is important to recognize that there are many different types of breaks or fractures, each with a different degree of severity.

— Green stick. (The bone is cracked, but not broken in two.)
— The simple fracture. (The bone is broken; the skin is not.)
— The compound fracture. (The bone and skin are broken in the same area.)
— The comminuted fracture. (The bone is shattered.)
— The separation of an epiphysis. (An end of the bone is broken away from the shaft. You will only see this in growing baby animals, not adults.)

The relatively mild green stick fracture is generally easily treated at home. All that is required is to keep the baby quiet, possibly with a light splint, for two weeks, until the bone has mended.

The simple fracture may be treated at home in some instances but, if at all possible, all the other fractures should be taken care of by a veterinarian. Even then, some fractures, such as the comminuted type, are difficult to treat.

UNDERSTANDING THE BROKEN LEG

In treating an animal with a broken leg, or just nursing it afterward, it is important to understand what has happened to the leg, and how to keep from doing further damage or dooming the animal by incorrect treatment, even if well meant.

When a leg is broken, often the muscles and ligaments tighten, which draws the ends of the bone into an overriding position. The leg must be stretched out, so that the ends of the bone are once again together. It is nearly impossible for a broken leg to heal when the bones are overriding. But you must be able to determine whether or not the pieces of bone *are* overriding, or if they are end-to-end. If you just pull away on a broken leg when the bones are end-to-end, you could do serious damage. Remember that you cannot simply put a cast or splint on a suspected broken leg! If the bones are overriding, you may be dooming the baby to a gangrenous limb and death.

TREATMENT OF A BROKEN LEG

PINNING

In many cases, the very best treatment for a broken leg is pinning, which your veterinarian must do for you. There are basically two types of pinning being done. The first, and most often used on infant animals, is the use of intramedullary pins. In intramedullary pinning, a stainless steel pin, *just large enough to fill the medullary cavity* (the hollow portion of the bone), is chosen. This pin is very strong and hard to bend or break. It is sharp at one end and often has a sharp, screw-threaded end on the other.

With the animal under sedation, the area over the break is clipped, then disinfected. An incision is made over the break, cutting down until both ends of the bones are visible. Any necrotic material, old blood clots or bone chips, are removed. Then the sharp, clean end of the pin is worked up through the bone shaft and out through the skin. Then the pin is inserted in the other end of the bone, with a special instrument, and the pin is screwed into the solid end of the bone. Care is taken not to go so far that the pin enters the joint or complications arise. For this reason, experience and a good X-ray machine are needed.

When the pin is firmly in place, the pin setter is removed from the end protruding from the skin, and the pin is cut off. There may or may not be a pin end remaining through the skin. Both heal well. There is seldom any need for extra support of the limb, and the baby will use the leg as before, as soon as the pain of the break subsides. Pinning is important to wild babies, as there is little restriction to their movement after the surgery, which keeps them from giving up, as sometimes happens when a heavy cast or splint are needed.

BONE PLATES

On occasion, especially with larger babies, it may be ncessary to use bone plating to immobilize a fracture. In bone plating, the fracture site is cleared, and a small stainless steel plate is placed over the break. Two or more stainless steel screws are then screwed into the bone on either side of the break, forming a sturdy bridge across the broken area. The reason that this method is not used as often as intermedullary pinning is that more extensive surgery is required to remove the plate, compared to very little surgery in the intermedullary pin. (In fact, often the pin can be unscrewed and removed without sedating the patient, with no discomfort to the animal.)

OTHER PINNING METHODS

There are two other pinning methods that are used to set broken legs, but they are very seldom used on baby animals, due to their small size. These methods are through-and-through pinning and the use of bone screws alone. Through-and-through pinning also needs a supportive plaster cast which frightens or depresses many babies, especially wild babies.

THE THOMAS SPLINT

This splint is often used when a bone cannot be pinned and there has been a complete break, making end-to-end alignment of the bone ends very necessary. The Thomas splint keeps steady traction on the broken leg, while providing support and protection.

A Thomas-type splint is fairly easy to construct at home and can be adapted to nearly every size baby. The splint can be made of wire, the gauge depending on the weight and the strength of the baby. A coat hanger will support a mild-mannered baby weighing 10 to 15 pounds. As the weight of the baby increases, so should the stiffness and gauge of the wire. A Thomas-type splint for a calf or foal can be made from lightweight pipe, welded by a local blacksmith, after measurements have been taken at home.

The Thomas splint acts both as a splint for the leg and a crutch for supporting the baby's weight. The circular portion of the splint should be large enough to encircle the top of the leg comfortably. Remember that the splint must be very well padded, so when measuring for the splint, make it large enough.

The splint wire can be held in form with adhesive tape. It will take a few try-ons before the size is correct. Use the unbroken leg, as too much handling of the broken leg may further damage it, and the fitting will cause discomfort to the baby. The splint is slipped over the leg and is positioned so that the lower portion of the round part of the splint fits snugly at the point where the leg and body come together. And, the splint should extend a short distance beyond the foot. If the round portion has not yet been padded, allow extra room.

Cotton can be used to pad the armpit rest of the splint. It should be quite thick, so there is no pressure from the wire. Such pressure will cause bad sores and also severe nerve damage. The cotton can be held in place with several wrappings of gauze, then tape. Be careful to get it very smooth. The smallest wrinkle can cause discomfort and sores.

Wide adhesive tape is cut so it will reach from the elbow (or above the hock) to eight inches below the foot. The tape should be wider than the leg so that when another matching piece is cut, they can completely encase the leg. The tape is used to put traction on the leg. When everything is correctly fitted, the tape is applied. It will stick very well if it is first sprayed with automobile starting fluid (ether). Be sure that when you spray you are ready to place the tape, as it will immediately become *very* sticky! And, one caution, *do not use the spray ether around any spark or open flame, as it is highly flammable!*

Put one piece on the underside of the leg, carefully keeping the leg straight. A helper is very useful. Smoothly press the tape down until there are no air pockets. Then place the top piece of tape. In many cases, the tape will completely enclose the leg and no more tape is needed. If the tape is not wide enough to *completely* enclose the leg, spiral a narrower piece of tape from elbow or stifle to the ankle. Don't cover the foot, as it will need to be exposed to check the circulation in the leg while the leg is in the splint. Be careful not to get the spiral strip of tape too tight, as it would restrict the circulation of the leg, possibly causing gangrene to set in.

Traction is applied, and the foot is pulled down to the bottom of the splint. The toes should almost, but not quite, touch the splint. If it does touch, the toes may become sore. If they just barely touch, you can pad the toes with a ball of cotton. If they do touch solidly, the splint is too short. The splint should not be too long, as the baby would not be able to handle it properly to walk on it.

When the right traction is arrived at (the leg should be stretched snugly, but not yanked on or overpulled), tie the tail ends of the adhesive tape below the paw securely to the foot of the splint.

With the break end-to-end and the leg in traction to hold it there, the splint is wrapped with wide adhesive, the entire length, to hold the leg in place. If this is not done, the leg could bow in or out, hampering healing.

In larger animals, very active ones, or in cases of severe breaks, it is a good idea to pad the leg well before the final wrappings of adhesive are applied.

The leg should be checked every day. There should be little swelling, and the exposed foot should remain warm to the touch. If it suddenly appears cold, contact your veterinarian at once, as this is the first sign of gangrene or impaired circulation.

If there has been a compound fracture, or if there are cuts on the broken leg, try to keep an air space around the area, even if you must cut small holes in the tape. Unless this is done, the area will weep serum and possibly pus, soon making the entire splint foul. With the air space, the broken skin will dry naturally and not become damp.

SIMPLE SPLINTS

Sometimes it is not necessary to provide traction for a broken leg. Some broken bones remain end-to-end and others, such as the green stick fracture, never completely break, but must have some additional support to prevent further breakage or injury.

In these cases, a simple splint is often adequate. A splint for a baby animal can be a ready-made aluminum spoon-type splint, a piece of stiff plastic, cardboard, or even Popsicle sticks. It must be strong enough to support the leg and the baby's weight. But, it must also be light enough to be handled by the animal.

The splint should be long enough to immobilize not only the broken section of the leg, but should extend from the toe to the uppermost joint on the leg. This type of splint is really not very good for breaks occurring between the hock and stifle, due to the natural angle of this area. If this area must be splinted, and a Thomas-type splint cannot be used, cut an angular splint out of very light plywood or heavy cardboard, so that the whole leg is immobilized.

To apply a simple splint, first pad the splint so that there are no sharp or hard edges to cause pressure. A light coat of cotton followed by a wrapping of gauze is generally acceptable. Lay the leg in the splint, being careful not to do damage to the leg. Then, with equal care, gently tape the splint in place. It is a good idea to spray the tape with automobile starting fluid (ether), as it makes the tape stick much better. Tape the leg in place snugly, but not tightly, as you may restrict the blood circulation and that can lead to gangrene.

It is a good idea to have a small area at the bottom open, so you can check the toes for coldness which signifies restricted circulation.

There is an inexpensive reusable cut-to-length padded light weight aluminum splint available that is very useful in bird and small animal babies with fractured legs. This is called a Sam splint and is available online and from many veterinarians. It works very well and is easy to use, as well as being comfortable to the wearer.

THE IMPORTANCE OF COMPLETE IMMOBILIZATION

Whatever type of treatment is used for a broken leg, there is great importance in having *total* immobilization of the limb. If there is movement in the area of the break, calcium may cover both broken ends of the bone, but will not bridge the break. The ending will be a false joint, leaving the leg nearly useless. With total immobilization, healing is generally complete in three weeks (small animals) to six weeks (larger ones).

BIRD LEGS AND WINGS

In general, a broken bone is a broken bone. When approaching the task of setting a broken leg or wing, first read the previous section on mammals. But there are many differences in the treatment of some broken bones in birds.

First of all, bird bones are very porous, which makes them light and easily broken. This lightness helps the bird to fly. The bones of mammals are more heavily constructed since they walk and run, but do not have to fly. In the same sense, birds that spend a lot or all of their time on the ground have heavier leg bones. A good example of

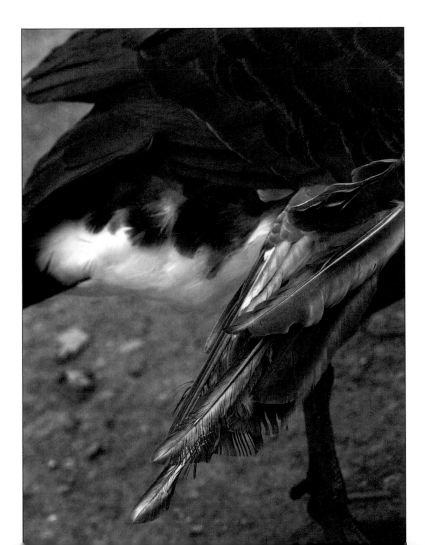

this is the ostrich, whose heavy leg bones give it the strength to run as fast as a horse.

Birds are also very uncooperative patients to nurse when they have broken bones. This is due, in part, to their natural tendency to try to escape what they fear and, in part, to their natural activity.

DIFFERENCES IN APPLYING THE THOMAS SPLINT

In birds, the Thomas splint is only practical when splinting a broken leg. The Thomas splint is much too clumsy for use on a wing, except in very rare instances.

We primarily use the Thomas splint on birds that prefer a standing position. Perching birds often fight the restriction and weight of it. It is very important in all birds to keep the weight and bulk of the Thomas-type splint down to the bare minimum needed to keep the correct traction on the leg, and to keep the splint from twisting. It is this occasional twisting, usually seen on long-legged birds, that makes sufficient support of the whole leg necessary. If twisting occurs, there will be movement in the break area, and either the bone will not heal or the bone ends may come out of alignment, possibly overriding.

When checking the toes of a bird wearing a Thomas-type splint, you must feel the bottom pads of both feet, as some bird's feet seem cool to the touch normally, and that could be mistaken for restricted circulation.

PINNING

Whenever possible, it is best to have a broken leg or wing pinned by your veterinarian. This gives very good and light support to the limb without bulk or a frightening contraption. There are very tiny pins which can be used on all but the very smallest baby birds.

The pins work very well on adult birds that have been injured by flying into wires, windows, or that have been shot by unthinking children with BB guns. Even with the more active adult, a pin usually helps the break heal within three weeks' time.

SIMPLE SPLINTS

Simple splints are used for many broken bones in birds. Here one has to use a little ingenuity, especially with wing breaks. Keep in mind the factors required for good healing of a broken bone:

1. Be sure the ends of the bone are end-to-end when the bone is splinted.
2. Be sure there is no movement in the broken part, or healing will not take place.
3. Be sure the leg is well supported by the splint, so no further damage can be done.

With these things in mind, try to devise an adequate splint that is light enough to be tolerated by the bird.

A few splinting materials that we have used from time to time include Popsicle sticks; tape, doubled or tripled; pieces of plastic, cut from dishwashing-liquid bottles; pieces of balsam wood (from hobby shops); and one-quarter-inch pine strips (often used to tack up plastic storm windows).

One caution: as in setting the bones of mammals, the job is much safer done by a veterinarian. He will know when the bones are end-to-end, and if the splint is in correct position. An inexperienced layperson can do unknowing damage.

When tape must be used in splinting a leg, a quick spray with automobile starting fluid (ether) will make the tape stick better. Caution: *Do not use this fluid near any open flame, as it is highly flammable.* You can again spray it when removing the tape, and the tape will come away without plucking or breaking the feathers. Any tape gum left on the feathers can be removed with a bit of the same fluid sprayed on a terry cloth.

After a wing is splinted, it is necessary to keep it inactive. One good way to do this is to enclose the bird in an old sock, just snug enough to restrict the wings without being too tight and doing further injury to the broken one. Just leave the head poking through a small hole in the toe and the feet through a slit in the bottom. The tail can be free, as well as the vent. Be sure to make the leg slit large enough to permit free movement, but not so loose that the bird will step on the surrounding area and shift the position of the sock.

Do not provide a perch for a bird with a broken limb because it will try to use the perch, probably falling, time after time. A solid-walled box with no "furniture" is much better.

Amputation
of Limbs

IT IS GENERALLY thought that any wild or domestic animal
or bird that suffers an injury to a limb so severe as to require amputation is better off "put out of its misery." We feel very strongly that this
is not true. Baby animals and birds, especially, seem to adapt very well
to the loss of a limb. Even wild babies often do very well minus a limb.
Even when it is not feasible to release a wild bird due to an amputation,
often it will do very well as a "semidomestic" neighbor. (Most animals
get along just fine with a leg missing, but some birds must have two feet
for grasping or swimming, or two wings for flying.)

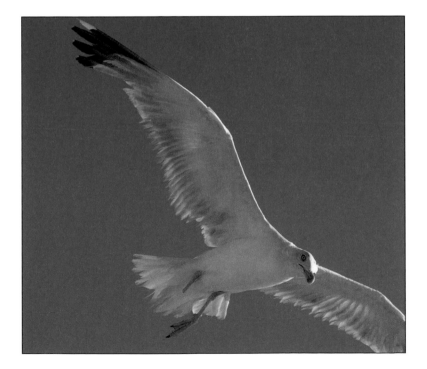

We have an amputee deer in the neighborhood, and it has lived through four hunting seasons and the worst winter in Minnesota history, without any human assistance at all!

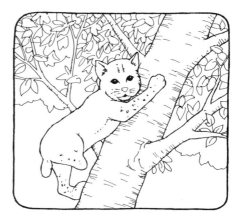

Wild cats can climb with three legs, a wolf can hunt, a deer run, and a bear forage. They need no pity, nor are they "ugly."

In fact, sometimes it is best to amputate a severely damaged limb rather than to put the animal through weeks of trauma trying to get the leg to mend. Your veterinarian can best advise you on this. *Do not try to perform an amputation yourself!* Not only is this cruel, but an amputation, when not done correctly, may have serious complications. In an amputation, you can't just "whack off" the limb!

Cuts

ON OCCASION, A baby animal is found suffering from some type of cut or tear. True, some such injuries should be sutured up, but seldom is the baby found before the injury is seriously contaminated with bacteria and debris. To suture such a wound is to invite serious infection. An alternate approach is usually taken. The wound is thoroughly flushed out with a mild, warm solution of Ivory soap and water. All noticeable foreign material is rinsed away, along with any blood clots and pus. Do be careful when rinsing away blood clots from a fairly fresh wound that has bled. With such a wound, there will generally be quite a bit of dried blood in the area. You won't want to start the bleeding again.

Trim all hair or feathers away from the immediate area, as they will mat over the sticky wound surface, retarding healing and inviting infection.

If the wound gapes open too badly, you can apply two or more butterfly bandages (see illustration) to help close the gap. But do not close it entirely. Leave the lowest area open so the wound can drain. Keep washing any seepage away and keep the wound coated with an antibiotic or sulfa powder. Do not use salve on cuts. It only attracts dirt and hair.

Where large areas of skin have been ripped away, soak the wound daily in a mild, normal saline solution, then apply a light antiseptic dressing. It should be an ointment that is not sticky or stiff, and that will keep the area soft and pliable. If absolutely necessary, a light gauze bandage may be applied to keep dirt out of the wound. *Do not bandage* if you can help it. Bandaged

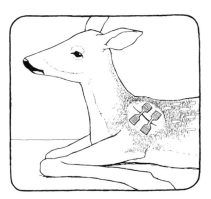

wounds on animals often become wet and putrid; wounds exposed to the air remain dry and heal quickly.

Animals that have had infected wounds should receive antibiotics or a sulfa for five days' time. This can be given by injection in bad infections where the animal is actually sick. Or it can be given in an oral form for preventative measures. The oral medication can be given in the food in most cases.

Gunshot Wounds

GUNSHOT WOUNDS ARE not as common in baby animals as they are in adults, but we have seen several babies with them. These wounds are usually suffered either at the hands of so-called hunters—who often are hunting out of season and shoot at anything that moves—or when a mother animal (often prowling in someone's chicken coop) is shot at, and one or more of her accompanying babies are hit.

SHOTGUN WOUNDS

Wounds caused by shot (which is the term used for the little BB's contained in a shotgun shell) are either fatal (close range), or cause injuries of varying degrees, depending on range and size of the shot. In wounds caused by shot, it is hard to see the place of entrance. Most shot is quite small, often smaller than a tiny pea. On entering the body, it does not expand much nor does it explode. Killing is caused by many pieces of shot entering different parts of the body. Often some strike a vital organ.

The animal must be examined very closely, under good light. Part the hair or feathers and examine the skin for tiny holes; often the holes are not even bleeding. The shot seldom needs to be removed, unless an X ray shows that a piece is in a dangerous area or is embedded in a vital organ. Generally, the body builds a coat of scar tissue around the shot, where it will remain for life.

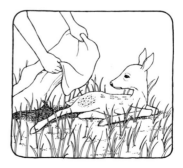

Shock is often seen. Keep the animal quiet and warm until it wears off. An injection of tetanus antitoxin, along with antibiotics for five days, is recommended. Keep all hair or feathers away from the entry holes, as they will close the holes over, encouraging infection.

RIFLE WOUNDS

Rifle wounds are often more serious than those inflicted by a shotgun. You will be able to tell them from other wounds by carefully peering into the opening in the skin, aided by a light. Usually, you will be able to see deep into the wound. Often, the bullet will have passed completely through the animal, so check not only for an entrance wound, but also an exit wound.

Rifle wounds are nothing to "play doctor" with. Take the animal to a veterinarian at once.

The animal will often be in shock (act listless, tremble, pant, and have pale mucous membranes), so keep it warm, and handle as little as possible.

STOPPING BLEEDING

Some wounds bleed severely, especially when a major blood vessel has been hit. This bleeding must be stopped quickly. If nothing is handy to use for a pressure bandage (a soft, absorbent cloth to press firmly on the wound), rip a section out of your clothes (shirttail, underwear, glove lining). Even pressure applied with bare fingers to a torn vessel is better than nothing.

Press the pressure pad very firmly on the area where the most bleeding is occurring. Often you can see the blood actually welling up from a small spot (the torn blood vessel). Press here. And, hold the pressure until the bleeding stops or you reach your veterinarian's office. Do not remove a cloth used as a pressure pack until your veterinarian tells you to, or until you are absolutely sure the bleeding has stopped completely. This is often the next day. If it is removed too soon, the bleeding may continue, and you might not be able to halt it a second time.

Small wounds that bleed profusely may be aided by applying powdered alum or a styptic powder. Both are common to most homes.

ADOPTING THE WILD BABY

If, for any reason, you decide to keep a wild baby you have rescued and fed by hand, please consider all aspects. There are, of course, some wild babies that cannot be released to the wild, as they would not survive. This includes all birds and animals that have suffered injuries that limit their hunting or foraging abilities. It also includes any animals that have been spoiled, taking away all natural distrust of man. To dump such an animal in the woods, without an actual release training period, is to condemn, it to certain death.

First, be sure you have a permit, enabling you to keep your wild baby permanently. We know of cases where wild babies, grown to adulthood, have been shot in the yard by game enforcement officers, due to illegal possession. Also, there are stiff fines for illegal possession of some wild animals.

Do not immediately declaw, de-scent, or defang a wild "pet." Such an animal cannot be released—ever. And, as its natural wild instincts arise at a later age, a time when you'll be living with it, you may wish you had not been so impetuous.

Keep in mind the animal's adult disposition. A cage is seldom the answer as a permanent home. Very few wild animals can stand close confinement. Visit another person with an adult animal of the same species you intend to keep. You can ask them how they get along with their wild pet. This will give you a pretty good idea as to whether you want to go through what they do. You cannot "own" a wild animal, though you can sometimes live with one.

When living with a wild animal, never think it is "tame," meaning domestic. It is not, and never will be. It may be docile, love attention, love children, and so on. But, when it feels threatened or is protecting its "own" food or its "own" territory (even if it is *your* roast or *your* couch), it will act like a "wild" animal, with no appreciation for the domestication you are imposing upon it.

You continually have to think about the animal's feelings in certain situations, and the animal's future reactions. Do this not only to protect yourself and those around you from accidents, but also to protect your relationship with the animal. Very few people can "out-bluff" a wild animal. Occasionally, people try to beat the "viciousness" out of an animal, but this measure is ignorant and cruel and only makes the situation much worse.

You will also have to think about your friends' and neighbors' reactions to your future pet. Will you lose friends because you are keeping a "dangerous" animal in your house, or because your house suddenly smells like a zoo? Be aware, too, that you will be held financially responsible for the actions of this pet, no matter how accidental an injury or damage may be. What seems like a small scratch to one person may appear to be a terrible wound to another!

After reading all this, you may decide that maybe the cute baby might best be raised with release in mind! We really hope so. Few people can survive happily in a relationship with an adult wild animal. It is so much better to raise the babies like you would your children. You love them, give them the best care you can while they need it, then you encourage them to be independent and let them go out on their own, with no strings attached.

And in the future, perhaps you will catch a glimpse of them in free adulthood, melting into a sun-dappled woods—and cry.

SECTION 5

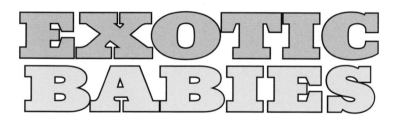

Monkeys

PERHAPS OF ALL the baby animals sold at pet shops, the little monkeys are the most adorable. Most monkeys sold for pets are quite young, as older monkeys are harder to tame and introduce into the home. It is the older monkey that often bites and screams at a touch. Many never do get tame enough to be a pet. So people who want a pet monkey are faced with raising an infant.

It is a very good idea to become familiar with monkeys *before* buying one. A monkey does make an interesting pet, but it is a demanding pet, requiring much time and care. *Before* buying that monkey, consider these facts:

— It is illegal in many states to own a monkey.
— Monkeys need a warm, draft-free room, even when caged. In temperatures below 70°F, a monkey will be prone to illness.
— Monkeys need a large cage. A two by two-foot parrot cage will *not* do. To be happy, an average size monkey needs a six by six by four-foot cage, built like a flight cage for birds.
— Monkeys seldom can be housebroken. When they have to go, they do—whether they are on the davenport or in Aunt Harriet's lap!
— Monkeys often bite when frightened, no matter how tame they are. And in some states any reported monkey bite results in a rabies exam or euthanasia.
— Monkeys are curious. Should one escape from the cage, it can just about wreck a room.
— Like people, monkeys get sick and require veterinary care from time to time.

Many different types of monkeys (and apes) are sold as pets. Some make good all-'round pets, some make good pets for a few especially understanding people, others do not make good pets for anyone.

Among the most common of the monkeys being offered for sale is the squirrel monkey. This small, wide-eyed monkey is fairly inexpensive and readily available. Unfortunately, it does not really make a good pet. The squirrel monkey is quite nervous by temperament and seldom very trusting of human beings. So, if you just want an active cage pet to watch and feed, the squirrel monkey is fine, but if you want a monkey you can handle and pet, one that will respond fully, you had better choose another species.

Another of the widely sold monkeys is the spider monkey. This is a very quiet, loving pet, but quite delicate. A small draft on this animal will often cause a slight indigestion, a fatal diarrhea, or other fatal illness. Excitement can cause a heart attack. A spider monkey can be a nice pet for someone with an evenly warm room for the cage and time to keep home conditions ideal. The spider monkey is one of the larger monkeys and requires a sizable cage to exercise in. If this is not provided, stiffness and arthritis can be a problem.

The capuchin, or organ grinder's monkey, is frequently a good choice for a pet. This is a medium-size, quite common monkey in the medium-price range. It is very intelligent and usually affectionate as a baby. Males are most often offered for sale but, unfortunately, the males have a tendency to become aggressive with age. Castra-

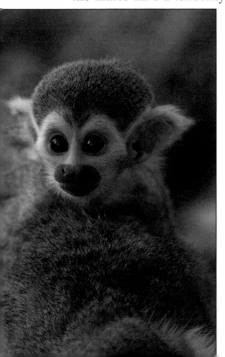

tion, before this becomes a problem, is a solution in many cases. All too often, though, an owner resorts to having the monkey defanged. This doesn't really solve anything, except to remove the physical danger of the teeth. The aggression is still there, the expression of it just changes form.

Capuchins often remain good pets as long as they receive enough exercise daily and minimal teasing or punishment. Teasing and punishment anger the monkey and frustrate it.

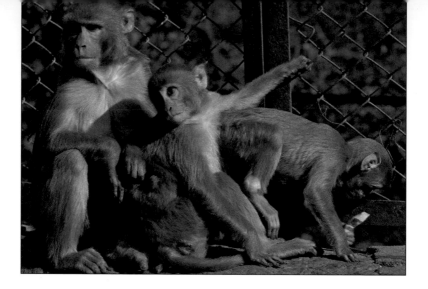

Some marmosets make fine pets in homes where there is little room for an exercise cage. Marmosets are small monkeys and are usually quite gentle. But, as with the squirrel monkey, because they are small, they are easily frightened by loud noises and quick actions.

If there is room for a large monkey, the rhesus monkey can be a nice pet. This is the monkey often used in laboratories to replace the human in tests. It is very intelligent and quite affectionate. But it is strong and quick, so it will need adequate exercise space and an understanding family. As it gets larger, it can become dangerous, if provoked.

Another large monkey is the macaque. This is a hardy monkey that adapts quite well in many homes. It too is very intelligent, so much so that it often outsmarts the people who own it!

Larger apes do not make good pets. Older animals, especially males become strong and aggressive; a dangerous combination for family life.

CHOOSING THE MONKEY

After reading all you can about different monkeys, it is a good idea to actually *see* the different species that are available to buy. One good place to start is at the nearest zoo. No, zoos do not sell monkeys to the public, but you will be able to see both juvenile and adults of many, many species. We think it is wise to see just how large some of these cute babies get, *before* buying one!

In actually shopping for the new baby, go to several breeders and actually see the monkeys firsthand. This will give you an idea of how young the monkeys actually are. A few breeders will offer older monkeys for sale instead of young ones. The stores can buy them cheaper and make a bigger profit by selling the older ones as young. These older monkeys may make fine cage pets, but seldom enjoy handling or close human contact.

Find out who sells the healthiest animals. Look for very clean cages. There should be no smell in the monkey area. Their food and water containers should be kept spotlessly clean and always full. Their coats should be shiny, not dull, nor full of dandruff and patchy. There should be no scabs or sores (other than a minor cut or scratch). Monkeys are like children and often have minor scrapes or scratches, but nasty-looking sores indicate a health problem.

DIET

It is best to read all you can on the type of monkey you have decided to buy. In this way, you will know not only what the pet shop has been feeding, but what the monkey's natural diet would be in the wild. In this way, you will best be able to stick close to a correct diet.

The diet of an older monkey, 10 months to a year or older, is usually quite easily formulated with the help of a special monkey food. But with the baby, there is room for more "mothering." Few baby monkeys will live if they must rely on a handful of dry monkey pellets placed in the cage. As with human babies, baby monkeys need a lot of attention.

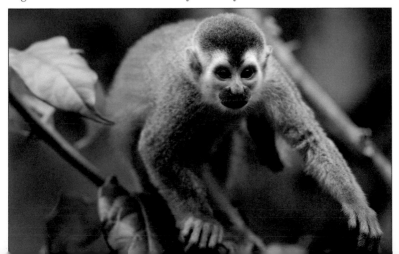

First of all, it is a good idea to get a good human pediatric liquid vitamin and see that the monkey gets it daily. This can be done by adding a drop or two to the water in most cases. But, once in awhile, you get a baby that dislikes the smell or taste. Who can blame them! In this case, you will have to give the drops by mouth, or possibly conceal them in a bit of fruit. If you can get away from fighting the baby over the vitamins, by all means do so. This small daily struggle can make that baby distrust you.

Monkeys do like fruit, but do not make the common mistake of only feeding bananas! There isn't enough nutrition in bananas alone, and eating too many bananas can cause digestive upsets. Remember that the monkey infant is tiny, so feed small bits of all kinds of fruit, and do not give too much of any one kind.

Hard-boiled egg yolks, boiled liver bits, small servings of good quality cat food (those little, fairly expensive cans), peanut butter on snack crackers, baby food, bread, small bits of both raw and cooked vegetables, and dry monkey biscuits will make up most of the diet. Very small portions of whole milk can also be given. But, don't overdo the milk. Diarrhea will surely result. Very young monkeys can be given milk, mixed with high-protein baby cereal, but too much liquid milk is not good.

WARMTH

Monkeys must be kept completely warm. Any small drafts can cause colds, pneumonia, and other illnesses. One way to keep the monkey comfortable is to provide a heat lamp in one corner of its exercise cage. The lamp should neither be in the cage, nor within the monkey's reach. Rather, it should be aimed through the wire at a resting shelf. The temperature in the resting area should be between 70° and 80°F. In this way the monkey, itself, can choose the most comfortable temperature.

The monkey's cage should not be situated in a room with an outside door, as there can be a draft in the room even in warm weather. A monkey does perfectly well outside in warm climates, provided that the temperature does not drop much at night. Damp, chilly days or nights quickly kill a monkey.

ILLNESS

As we have noted, monkeys are susceptible to many of the diseases that humans are, including the common cold. But monkeys are much smaller than humans and do not have the stamina that humans do. Thus, a cold can quickly turn into pneumonia, or a minor ailment into a fatal one.

Be sure to check your monkey daily. Note the consistency of his droppings, his breathing, and both eye and nasal mucus. Also notice his appetite, activity, and water consumption. Any deviations from normal should be regarded with suspicion.

Symptoms of sickness are: runny nose or eyes, swollen eyelids, coughing, droopiness, lack of appetite, diarrhea, or constipation.

It is a good idea to put on a pair of heavy leather gloves when handling a sick monkey, as sick monkeys are often crabby and do not like to be handled. Take the temperature, rectally. Then call your veterinarian. It is a very good idea to have recorded your monkey's normal temperature on a day soon after it was brought home and appeared well. There is a variation of temperatures among monkeys, with smaller species running a higher normal temperature than larger ones.

The monkey should be carried to the veterinarian's office in a small, sturdy cardboard box or a small cat carrier. A frightened monkey does not make a pleasant companion in the car while you are driving in rush-hour traffic!

Tuberculosis is quite common in monkeys, so it is a good idea to have your monkey checked yearly, even when it appears healthy. This is a simple test, done by your veterinarian, and only involves a tiny bit of tuberculin serum being injected into the skin of the monkey's eyelid. The eyelid is examined 72 to 96 hours later for signs of redness and swelling, indicating a positive reaction.

Coatimundis

THE COATIMUNDI, OFTEN called a coati, is quite similar to a raccoon, with the exception of its long, upturned nose and long, less bushy tail. These animals are often found in the Southwest, more or less replacing the raccoon in this area. They range mainly in the daytime, but are also found at night in some instances. They are also raised in pens for sale by breeders. The babies make very nice pets and are not so terribly snoopy the way baby raccoons are. As they mature, coatimundis can become aggressive, so they should be treated with respect from infancy. As with monkeys, it is best to buy only a young coati, if you are determined to own one. Keep in mind that they do require a large cage and plenty of attention to be a good pet. They are inquisitive and are not easy to house-train.

Be sure to get only a healthy baby that has been well-cared-for. Baby coatis must be kept in a clean, dry pen, with both food and water available to them while in the pet shop. Dirty pens, smelly cages,

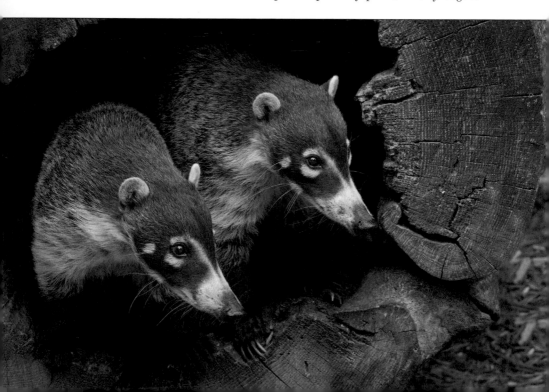

and empty food and water dishes are signs that the breeder could use better help or management. Buy elsewhere.

The baby coati itself should have a shiny coat and look bright. It may be a little shy, but should not snarl and snap when a hand is placed into the cage.

Always make sure it is legal in your state to own a coati.

DIET

Baby coatis are quite easy to feed. They have a wide variety in their natural diet. Very tiny coatimundis can be fed similarly to baby raccoons. They are a little rough on bottle nipples, however. If they are able to handle it, a small lamb nipple often works better than a pet nurser nipple, as it is longer and much stronger.

At about six to seven weeks of age, coatis begin taking large quantities of food, other than milk. At this time, some very good first foods for them are: a good quality canned dog or cat food, hardboiled egg yolk, small portions of raw vegetables, fruit, and dry dog food chunks, soaked in milk.

At first, the babies are quite messy when fed, but they soon quickly eat what is offered, with less playing and investigating.

As the baby coati begins eating more and more solid food, taper off the liquid milk fed. If offered, the baby will drink huge quantities of milk, but soon will begin suffering from digestive upsets.

COMMON ILLNESSES

DIARRHEA

Diarrhea is usually caused by overfeeding, especially too much milk. At the first sign of diarrhea, cut back the food given at the next feeding. Do keep water available at all times as dehydration can quickly be a problem. In simple cases of diarrhea, caused by a slight digestive upset, just cutting down the amount fed for two feedings brings about a quick halt to the diarrhea. If this does not help, give the baby coati 6 to 12 cc of kaolin-pectin (depending on his size). Repeat this every two hours until relief is noticed. If this does not work within 6 to 10 hours (again, depending on size), remove all solid food and milk from the diet and replace it with an oral electrolyte solution. If the diarrhea progresses for some time, the baby begins to dehydrate. In dehydration, the coati loses not only body fluids, but also essential body salts and chemicals. These must be replaced, or it will die. The oral electrolytes provide fluid, electrolytes (body salts and chemicals), and also a little nutrition which can be absorbed.

Should the baby appear weak or not recover promptly from the diarrhea, contact your veterinarian at once. He may need to administer antibiotics or injectable electrolytes.

DISTEMPER

Coatimundis are susceptible to both canine and feline distemper. Symptoms include lack of appetite, diarrhea, depression, and mattered eyes. Reputable breeders keep all their stock vaccinated but, if in doubt as to your new baby coati's vaccination status, it is best to revaccinate. Your breeder often will have health papers available for the babies, and recorded on this should be the date of vaccination and the name of the product used. Jot this information down, then talk to your veterinarian. Sometimes coatis are only vaccinated for canine distemper but, as they are susceptible to feline distemper, protection for both is necessary.

After the first injection, a booster soon after is required; then yearly boosters are required for full protection.

RABIES

Unfortunately, rabies is quite common in wild coatimundis. This is *the* prime reason for choosing a pet coati from pen-raised animals, instead of wild-caught coatis. The rabid coati is not necessarily the furious, "mad" animal depicted in movies. They often are very loving, or just very quiet. A person need not even get bitten to contract the disease.

Contact with the rabid coati's saliva is enough—and few people bother having a dead pet coati checked for rabies if no one was bitten by it.

The pet coati should be vaccinated yearly with an inactivated rabies vaccine not just for the coati's protection, but for the protection of the whole family.

GENERAL CARE

Adult coatis are easily cared for, but they do need some attention. They make a nice house pet, but trash containers and lower cupboards must be "coati-proofed." Extra care needs to be taken to house-train them. At first, try placing baby coati in a large box, with a litter pan at one end, away from its favorite "nest" corner. It will usually choose one spot for its toilet, and you can put the litter pan in that spot. Leaving one or two droppings in the pan may help it learn what the pan is for. *Do not* punish the coati for "accidents," but do clean up any spots well with bleach water or strong soap to eliminate any odor that might draw it back to the wrong spot.

It is best to have your young coati spayed or neutered as it will prevent a lot of aggressive, territorial behavior in the future.

Adult coatis are easily fed, doing well on a basic diet of dry dog food, with additions of monkey chow, fruit, canned meat, vegetables, and hard-boiled eggs. They are best fed twice daily, with water available at all times. Coatis have a tendency to root and dig, so use heavy crocks for food and water containers to avoid spills and mess.

Be sure that the coati has a "private" spot where it can go and curl up for a nap without disruptions. Many people are bitten when a slightly crabby coati is aroused from its nap.

Coatimundis do well in an outdoor pen during warm weather. Do remember that coatis are warm-climate animals, so do not leave them out in damp, cool weather. To do so is condemning the coati to death. They are strong animals, with a tendency to dig, so be sure that the pen is sturdily constructed with heavy gauge two by four-inch wire, buried at the bottom.

Tamanduas

IN OUR OPINION, the tamandua, also known as the lesser anteater, is one of the nicest of house pets, provided a person is willing to take a little trouble with a pet. Tamanduas are fairly expensive; expect to pay the equivalent of the cost of a registered dog. . .or more, from a reputable breeder. The tamandua is a plushy, medium-size animal that loves people! It is sort of like a live toy. Tamanduas do not bite, as they have no teeth available for biting, nor the inclination to do so. Their only defense is their huge front claws, which are used to open logs and anthills. An aggressive or frightened anteater will raise up on its hind legs, holding its formidable clawed arms out in an attitude of defense. Before considering a tamandua for a pet, be absolutely sure that it is legal in your state and city; some forbid owning exotic animals.

As we have said, the tamandua does have a few requirements that some people may not be able to meet. The tamandua comes from

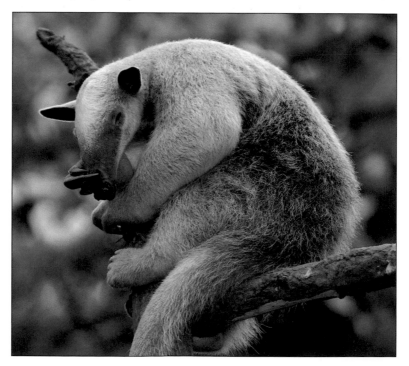

warm climates in South America, so remember, if you buy one, that it needs a stable, warm, draft-free environment at home. It also needs to be respected and not be overhandled. Overhandling kills many tamanduas. Perhaps this is because they are so "huggable." But it must be remembered that the tamandua is a wild animal, regardless of its apparent docility, and emotionally, wild animals are not up to a lot of well-meant handling.

And, finally, we come to the tamandua's diet. The tamandua is one animal that doesn't adapt to a ready-made diet as it lives basically on ants and grubs in nature. Its whole body is made up to survive best on this diet, from the long snout and long tongue to the huge, strong, front claws.

DIET

A tamandua's diet must be prepared daily, as it does not like "old" food. And a mixture it is, though no contents of the diet are exotic (such as South American ants) or expensive. The tamandua does well on a mixed food, but it must be supplied often, as it eats frequently, taking small quantities at a time. A tamandua cannot be fed one feeding daily and do well.

The mixture for the tamandua's diet is as follows:

    2 hard-boiled eggs

    ¼ pound finely ground meat (beef, liver, kidney)

    ¼ pound high-protein dry dog food

    1 ounce high-protein dry baby cereal

    ½ cup raw chopped spinach.

Add enough whole milk to make the mixture into a gruel consistency. Mix very well, leaving very few lumps or dry spots. A blender works beautifully! Then, just before feeding, add a few drops of lemon juice or vinegar. The tamandua seems to love the tart lemon juice, perhaps because ants are tart in taste.

Do not feed the tamandua cold food, straight from the refrigerator. The food should be brought to room temperature. This can be done by placing a cup with the food in it in a bowl of hot water, until the food is warmed. *Do not* leave the food out on the counter for long periods to warm up. This can cause the growth of dangerous bacteria, causing serious digestive upsets or death due to food poisoning.

GENERAL CARE

The tamandua is quite easy to care for, providing its simple needs are met. But the tamandua should not be allowed unsupervised access to the house. They like dark holes and crevasses, often getting into trouble by entering such places. For instance, they will crawl down an open register or heat duct, under a refrigerator, or under the floor. And, for some reason, either they don't remember how they got there, or are too confused to get out the way they came in. We once had to tear up the living room floor when a pet tamandua decided to enter a register he'd pried open!

It is much safer to provide the tamandua with a large, strong cage to protect it whenever supervision is not possible. This cage must be large enough for it to get adequate exercise when alone, but it must not become a jail cell.

The tamandua is quite resistant to most common diseases found in cats and dogs, but it does get ill from time to time. It is best to take its temperature when first brought home, and weekly thereafter for three weeks. Record this normal temperature to use as a guide. Should the animal appear depressed, lose its appetite, or show any other sign of illness, take the temperature immediately. If it is at all elevated, contact your veterinarian at once.

Skunks

SKUNKS, ANOTHER TYPE of "wild" baby commonly sold for a pet in many pet shops, often make a good house pet. One caution; *do not catch a wild baby skunk* with the idea of keeping it for a pet. The reason for this is *not* the problem of de-scenting the skunk, but a much more serious problem—rabies. Rabies is quite common in wild skunks in many areas. Even very young baby skunks can come in contact with these rabid skunks and become carriers of the disease. Rabies may incubate in a carrier for up to a year or longer before the animal shows symptoms of the disease, possibly infecting one or more humans long after it has become a pet, or even after it has received a rabies vaccination.

Pen-raised skunks are usually vaccinated yearly, do not come in contact with wild animals, and are quite safe as pets. They are also de-scented at a very young age. It is a nasty and smelly job to try to de-scent an older baby skunk, so this, in addition to the rabies problem, is why very few veterinarians will de-scent skunks brought in from the wild. Remember that once a skunk has been de-scented, it is helpless and can never be set free.

Skunks adapt well to living in the home and are generally easily housebroken. Although they are mainly nocturnal in the wild, skunks

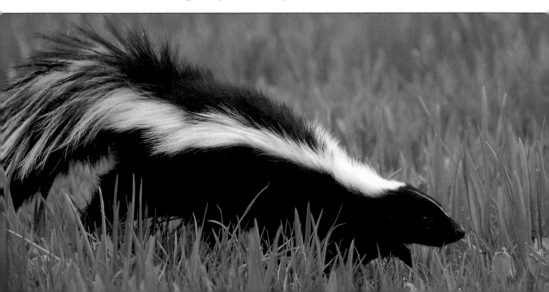

often become more active in the home during the daytime, making them more enjoyable as pets.

CHOOSING THE PET SKUNK

Many pet shops carry baby skunks in the spring, or can order one for you from a reputable breeder. These baby skunks are generally from six to nine weeks old. At this age, the babies are weaned, but not yet independent. Many baby skunks are nervous when first handled, but avoid a skunk that acts savage, snarling and stamping at every noise or motion. Both male and female skunks make good pets, so the sex of your pet should not matter, unless you intend to breed. Just try to pick out a bright-eyed, clean, shiny baby, with a quiet disposition.

DIET

Skunks are very easily fed. Very young babies should be fed several times daily, giving small feedings. Baby skunks do well on a variety of nutritious foods. The basis for their diet should be a good quality dry puppy food. In addition, small portions of these foods may be given: baby food, cooked and raw vegetables, cooked and raw meat (no highly spiced or fried meat), fruit, and hard-boiled or baked eggs. Milk may be used to moisten the puppy food, but do not give large quantities of liquid milk, or the baby will probably get diarrhea.

As the baby grows, you may cut down the frequency of the feedings, gradually increasing the size of each meal. The baby should be fed enough to keep in good flesh and growing in size and weight, but not overfed. Baby skunks can eat so much, if allowed, that they bloat and can die.

GENERAL CARE

Skunks are generally quite healthy, provided they receive proper care and regular vaccinations to protect them against common diseases to which they are susceptible. For example, skunks are susceptible to both canine and feline distemper, as well as to rabies, just like dogs and cats. They should be vaccinated regularly by your veterinarian to protect them against all three. Remember, skunks should receive only inactivated or killed vaccine to protect them against rabies.

As with dogs and cats, skunks should have an examination by a veterinarian twice a year for internal parasites. If necessary, they can receive medication which will kill any internal parasites that may be present. Do not just go ahead and buy worm medicine from your local store and worm them, without knowing if they have worms or what kinds of worms are present. To do this is to invite trouble as all worm medicine is toxic, and some is very dangerous.

If the skunk begins to scratch itself, examine its coat for fleas or lice. Look very carefully, as both of these mites are very small. Should you find anything suspicious, dust the skunk well with a flea powder. Use one meant for cats, as these products are usually safest. A powder containing rotenone is quite safe, even if the skunk should lick some from his coat.

Skunks are sensitive to many common household cleaners, such as Lysol, so use care to rinse floors well if such products are used. Sometimes a skunk picks up harmful chemicals on its feet, then licks them off while eating. Convulsions and unconsciousness can result in some instances.

Adult skunks can be fed once daily a mixture of dry dog food, good quality canned dog food, vegetables, fruit and meat. They will also, if given free run of the house, consume many mice. Our skunks have been better mousers than our cats! One caution, though: if the skunk does run free in the house, *don't use rodent baits or poisons.*

Armadillos

ARMADILLOS ARE COMMON in the southern regions
of the United States and are sold in some pet shops. The armadillo
can make an interesting and undemanding pet. They are also quite
inexpensive exotics. Their natural diet consists of grubs, insects, and
insect eggs. The normal range in the United States is the South, but
different species are found in Mexico, and Central and South America.
However, they are illegal to own in some states, so before you buy a pet
armadillo, check into this or face a fine.

The armadillo is a quiet animal in nature, and it is quite content
to shuffle along in its daily foraging expeditions. It looks like a cross

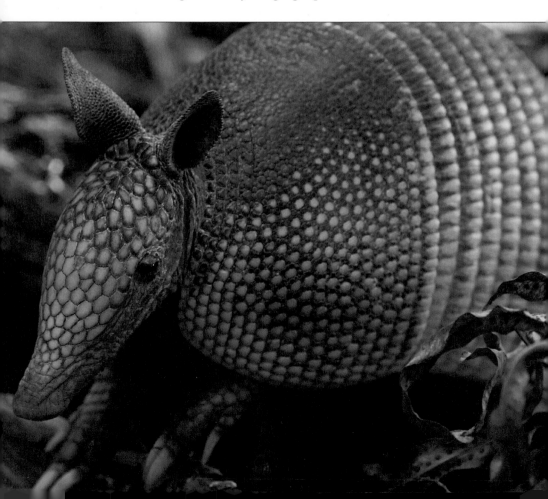

between a tank and an animated toy. The armadillo is similar to the anteater in that it is a pleasant pet and lives mainly on insects. Both have strong front claws, meant to dig insects from logs and nests, and both have long tongues, meant to slurp up soft foods. Neither has teeth capable of biting people.

But for all its good qualities, it is only fair to mention the less desirable traits. First of all, the armadillo is not an intensely affectionate pet. It is also not really "bright" by human standards. The armadillo cannot be left free in the house as it will rummage throughout the house, tipping over wastebaskets, rumpling rugs, and even knocking over light furniture.

DIET

Armadillos are quite easy to feed. They will thrive on a mixture which has been recommended for tamanduas. Or, they can be fed a mixture of good quality canned dog food, pabulum, and milk. Remember that a good quality canned food contains meat as a primary ingredient—not cereal by-products.

This food—at room temperature—should be fed at least twice daily. It should not be allowed to dry out or become spoiled. The food can be fed out of a shallow, heavy rabbit crock to prevent spills. (Armadillos are clumsy feeders and *very* pronc to tipping over dishes.)

A little lemon juice, mixed with honey, is a great treat for them. Of course, it should not be overdone.

HEALTH

In general, the armadillo is quite hardy. It should be housed in a room of at least 70°F with no drafts; otherwise chilling and pneumonia will become a serious problem.

Injuries kill many armadillos. Just because they appear heavily armored, with hard backplates, some people have a tendency to handle them harshly. Never drop the armadillo, or let a dog "play" with one to see it curl up in defense. The armadillo's shell can be punctured, and the nonarmored portions of its body are easily injured.

It is a good idea to have a yearly parasite examination done by a veterinarian. Armadillos seldom have many internal parasites, but in captivity the chances increase as their ranging area is limited.

GENERAL CARE

Armadillos are easily cared for, requiring only a moderate-size exercise cage and good handling. The cage should be strongly constructed to contain the animal, and to protect it from dogs and well-meaning children.

The cage should be in a room of at least 70°F to protect the armadillo from chill and drafts.

The armadillo *loves* water and will appreciate a swimming "pool" even if it is only a plastic dishpan. Remember to provide safe entrance and exit from any such pool. If a pool is not available, put a few inches of tepid water in the bathtub, and let it wade and splash to its heart's content. This animal is an excellent swimmer, using swimming to evade natural predators. It can even swim underwater. But don't just throw it into a full tub of water. Accidents can happen, and an armadillo *can* drown. It will be just as content to splash and wade around.

Its love of water often makes water dish spills inevitable. Use a very heavy crock, wedged well into a corner of the cage for as much protection as possible.

A special treat for the armadillo is to forage for its "own" meals. This can be done by providing access to your backyard, or even bringing a few grubs or a chunk of sod indoors. Be *very* careful that the grubs and sod are not taken from an area that has been sprayed or dusted with an insecticide or herbicide. Both can kill the armadillo.

Pet Shop and Humane Society Babies

PUPS and KITTENS

THERE IS A special feeling that comes from bringing home an animal from a pet shop or humane society. Maybe it is because that one animal was chosen from so many others and was the one that appealed most to *you*, personally! But this feeling can quickly disappear unless the ownership is backed with a little knowledge.

BEFORE BRINGING THAT PUP OR KITTEN HOME

Get at least one good booklet on care and training. Puppies do not come home and immediately turn into well-mannered guests. At first the pup will be nervous and lonely, and it will probably whine, howl, and have a few accidents. Punishment at this stage can permanently destroy a potentially good relationship. It is better to understand the puppy fully and plan for its actions. Have a few inexpensive toys for the pup to chew on and play with that will be its *own*. A heavy bone (that cannot be eaten or splintered), a

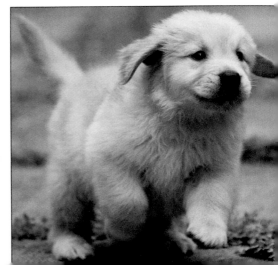

rawhide chew toy and a rubber ball (which, again, cannot be eaten) make good toys. Don't give a puppy an old shoe or sock to play with, as it might mistake a newer one for its toy. It won't be easy for the pup to understand why it can play with one shoe or sock, but is punished for playing with another.

Have a box in a private location for the puppy's *own* bed. At first, it is a good idea to keep puppies in one room only. That room should have an easily washable floor, such as linoleum or tile. House-training will be much easier this way. Lay a good layer of papers at the opposite end of the room from the bed. Puppies do not like to dirty their bed area, and naturally head toward the papers to answer nature.

If the pup is taken outdoors after each meal, it will soon become housebroken, painlessly.

Likewise, kittens do not just come into a strange house and instantly use the litter pan. For the first week or two, expect a few accidents, and work to prevent them—but don't punish for them. Keep the kitten in one room, containing its litter pan, unless the kitten is closely supervised. And do not change the tray daily—until the kitten uses it without fail. You can remove any really smelly contents, as a kitten's nose is much better than yours. But it needs a little smell to draw it to the box and act as a reminder of its use. If it is reeking of waste, the kitten won't go near it. Instead, the kitten will probably go under your bed or in the closet. Once formed, this kind of habit is terribly hard to break!

CHOOSING THE PUP OR KITTEN

It is very important to give a lot of thought to just what you want in a pet, and then to choose a pet that closely fits your needs. Don't buy that cute, adorable St. Bernard pup when you have a little yard or live in an apartment, thinking that you can walk it every day. Somehow, many people quickly tire of that daily routine. Remember that *every* day includes during blizzards, sweltering hot days, rainy days, and days you want to have a special "away from home" day.

If you are usually away from home all day, you might better consider a cat, as its needs are simpler than a dog's and cats seem to get along fine when left to their own devices all day. Dogs have a tendency to chew, dig, howl, and "potty" to let the frustrations they feel at being "abandoned" by their people. Cats tend to be more independent.

Read about the different breeds of both dogs and cats. You should have an idea what each one is like, and how each might fit into your life and fill your needs. We are not saying that you should buy or adopt only a purebred, but studying the breeds will give you an idea of what to expect, even in mixed breeds.

HEALTH

Now we come to, perhaps, the most important disadvantage of buying a pup or kitten from a pet shop, or bringing one home from a humane society, the possibility of the baby's having come into contact with a sick animal. No matter how well-cared-for the babies are, *no one* can tell when a pup or kitten is *about* to come down with a contagious disease. True, an experienced person can often spot early symptoms, but no one can anticipate the trouble *before* symptoms appear.

Thus, a sick pup can pass on its bacteria or virus to its litter-mates. Then they can pass it to other pups in the same pen, and so on. Even if the pups are vaccinated against the disease they are incubating, they may still well come down with the disease, regardless of the vaccination.

When one gets a pup or kitten from such a source, one can never be certain it will remain healthy, but there are a few things that will help cut the odds against trouble. First of all, get that pup or kitten from a well-run shop or shelter. Some shelters are very dirty. The dogs are wet and ill-kempt. There is a very foul odor about the place all the time (most kennels have some odor, unavoidably, but there should not be a foul stench about the place). Food is dumped on the ground or in a single community container. The building is quite dark and cluttered by food bags, cans, or other trash. But, to the other extreme, there are very clean shelters which are well managed, not overcrowded, and well lit.

In the same way, some pet shops are nasty, to say the least. We have been in some where animals were practically dying of thirst. Bird cages had no seed, but only a dish full of hulls, blown about by the bird's frantic begging for food and water.

Puppies in small, often foul cages and no exercise pen also indicate a badly run pet shop.

The pups and kittens from the ill-run shelter or shop may live and make very good pets—but they might die in a week or two from a severe infectious disease as well.

Never accept a pup or kitten with: diarrhea, mattered eyes, runny nose, or indications of skin trouble (red skin, baldness, or scabs). Such an animal is showing symptoms of distemper, pneumonitis, or possibly mange. All can be very serious diseases and hard to cure.

It is not a good idea to accept a baby from the same pen as the sick one is in, or one nearby. All these diseases can be very contagious. A well-run shop or shelter will not leave an animal that shows these symptoms among other animals that are well. However, a few badly run establishments will, often due to ignorance.

All babies should have had their first distemper vaccinations, and you should see written proof of it. *Do not just take the person's word.* See it on paper, signed by a veterinarian, not just the manager. In this way, you will know that your new pet has received the best protection possible. Be sure you take the pet to your own veterinarian for a checkup soon after bringing it home, and plan to return in time for the needed booster shot. It is also a good idea to have the new baby checked for the presence of internal parasites before you take it home. Worms and coccidiosis are common in confined pups and kittens. If they are quickly eliminated, they do not cause trouble in most cases. But if these pests are left to multiply, they can kill the baby in a short time.

SECTION 6

APPENDIX

Shelter for Disabled Birds

FLIGHT CAGES

A FLIGHT CAGE is often a necessary structure. Because it must be large enough to allow the bird that occupies it to fly about, the size and construction depend largely on the type of birds it will hold.

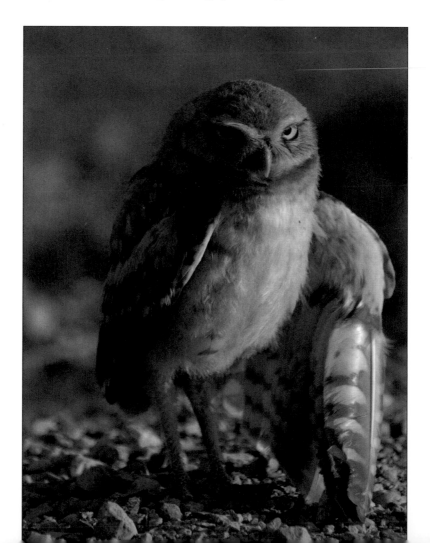

By "fly about" we do not mean merely that the bird can flit from one perch to the other, but that it can actually fly.

Such a cage can have many uses, ranging from permanent housing for handicapped birds to temporary housing for "teenage birds"—those old enough to leave the nest, but not old enough to feed themselves or survive in the wild. We have also used flight cages to house the babies of mammals before they were old enough to survive releases.

A permanent flight cage for small to medium-size birds can be inexpensively constructed, using one-half-inch hardware cloth stapled to one by four-inch furring strips. The one by four-inch furring strips need not have mitered corners, but can be made very sturdy by using L-shaped corner braces and corner clips (which have many sharp teeth, bridging the corner and lending strength).

Outdoor cages are best anchored by using four by four-inch posts at the corners; otherwise, high winds or some accidental misuse might tip them over.

A person need not have extraordinary carpentry skills to construct the flight cage, nor are expensive tools required. A very large cage can be made, using nothing more than a handsaw, hammer, tape measure, level, square, and a pair of wire cutters or tin snips—all tools commonly found in most homes.

All flight cages should be high enough to allow a human adult to enter and walk around without stooping over. This makes catching birds, cleaning the cage, and daily feeding and watering chores much easier.

For larger birds, especially larger birds of prey, the hardware cloth may not be strong enough. Instead, you may wish to use chain link fencing.

It is easiest to make the flight cage in sections, doing all the wire cutting and stapling on the flat ground, which will lend extra support. It seems that when you try to work on the framework after it is in place, it quickly becomes flimsy and easily broken.

Be sure that the cage is totally enclosed, with no tiny cracks or places where the wire *almost* joins. Such places are sure to cause injuries and fatalities. It seems that the birds are drawn to them.

They get stuck partway through and do serious injury to themselves in the frantic panic they feel in trying to escape.

All wire ends should be stapled securely to wood, leaving no pockets, bulges, or cracks.

Outdoor flight cages need protection from high winds, rain, and hot sun. This can be partly supplied by topping the cage with a water-proof roof and adding a "storm shelter" in a corner. This storm shelter can be a shed-type enclosure open to the south, but giving protection from the other three directions. It should have a perch large enough for comfortable resting, and high enough to make resting there comfortable to the bird.

The cage itself should have at least three inches of good, clean, coarse sand on the bottom to eliminate dampness or to keep puddles from forming in wet weather. Nothing kills birds easier than chill and dampness.

A flight cage should have at least two good perches. These can be tree branches with most of the smaller twigs trimmed off. Clean branches of this type are easier to *keep* clean, as the small twigs are not there to hold the droppings. Be sure that the size of the perches are right for the birds housed in the flight cage. A large bird cannot rest comfortably grasping a small branch, and a small bird needs a small perch or lameness may result.

A simple way to supply water, both for bathing and drinking, is to use a rectangular cake pan, buried in the sand bottom of the cage. Then put an inch-and-a-half of water in the pan. If small birds are to use it, it is safest to place several flat stones in one end of the pan, to act as steps in getting out of it. If these "steps" are not there, very small birds could drown if they are not able to climb out of their "pond."

The water must be changed daily. If this is not done, the water soon becomes foul—a perfect breeding ground for bacteria.

The sand on the bottom of the cage does not need to be cleaned daily, but should definitely be cleaned as soon as accumulations of droppings are noticed under favorite perches. Do not wait for them to pile up. This invites parasitic and bacterial infections.

While most flight cages are seen outdoors, it may be desirable or necessary to build indoor flight cages. We think that indoor flight cages are the ultimate in home decoration. Even pet birds, such as parakeets and canaries, *love* the freedom of a big flight cage. (We've never seen really happy pet birds in small cages!)

The indoor flight cage can be placed in just about any spot in the house, so long as it is warm and dry. Many people include a flight cage in their living room. Such a cage can be furnished with living plants, a waterfall, or whatever stirs your imagination. The main requirement is for a safe, warm, dry, and spacious place for recuperation or growing.

Many people prefer an indoor flight cage in place of the outdoor cage. It may be because there are many free-roaming cats, dogs, and children in the area and an outside flight cage can be quickly destroyed by them. Or, perhaps the people have decided to keep a rescued bird that has a permanent handicap, making release an impossibility.

The indoor flight cage is built along the same lines as the outdoor cage. Sand is also used on the floor of the indoor flight cage. Not only is it the easiest material to keep clean, but it is usually dust-free and dry at the same time. Sawdust can be used for the same purpose, but it will cause dust in the house.

Be sure that there is adequate lighting in the flight cage. If no natural light is available, as from a window, it is necessary to provide at least one lamp. We have had good luck using those clamp-on bed lamps with a flexible neck. We clamp them onto the top, outside of the cage, flexing the lamp to shine in through the wire. Placing a lamp inside the cage is unwise, as birds will often perch on it, causing a possible fire hazard.

HOUSING FOR WATERFOWL

Waterfowl that are disabled, either temporarily or permanently, have certain "special" requirements. First off, nearly all waterfowl are *messy* to keep. The birds love to flap, splash, and be extravagant with water. Of course, this water might be a pond or pool, but it might also be their water dish! We've had a wounded goose that tried to take a bath in our toilet bowl and a mallard that decided our 55-gallon aquarium would make a nice pond—complete with tasty "minnows." (The "minnows" were our highly prized Delta guppies—some costing more than $15 a piece!)

Any kind of slippery floor is out, be it linoleum or smooth concrete. Birds tend to slip and slide around, often severely spraining legs or doing other serious injury to themselves.

And daily exercise is a must both for rehabilitation of temporarily disabled birds and for those that have permanent handicaps, which prevent their release. Nothing is sadder than to see a beautiful water bird living in a small pen. Such a bird seldom lives long. It seems like they just aren't happy and pine away.

It's best for water birds to be housed outdoors in the summer, then moved to a more sheltered house for the winter unless, of course, you live in an area with very mild winters and little or no snow.

Again, a reminder: if you are going to keep a bird, be sure to contact your game warden. Many birds are protected, and you could get into trouble by keeping one illegally. It's safest to check and thereby to avoid unpleasantness!

A SUMMER OUTDOOR YARD

Water birds do best in large, well-drained outside pens during all moderately warm months (25°F and above). Simple construction of such an outdoor yard for them will take the average family or person about one day.

MATERIALS

1. One or more rolls of 2 by 4-inch welded wire, 6 feet high. Measure the outside dimensions of the yard, and you will know how much wire you will need. Be sure the pen is large enough! A single duck will need at least a 5 by 10-foot pen and

a heron a 20 by 20-foot pen. Birds that fly can use double these measurements.

2. Four by four-inch wood fence posts, at least seven-and-a-half feet long, one for every foot of line fence, or one at each corner.

    These posts should be cedar, tamarack, or another long-lasting wood. As long as you are building a fence, you might as well make one that will last!

3. A pair of tin snips.

    Wire cutters will do, but the tin snips are much faster.

4. A pound or more (depending on size of yard) of regular fence staples.

    Poultry netting staples will not do, as larger water birds can pop them out if they hit the fence.

5. Enough two by four-inch boards to go around the top of the yard.

    This strengthens the wire and gives something to tack the top wire onto.

6. Enough poultry netting to cover the top two-inch mesh in at least four-foot rolls.

    This netting is not only to prevent birds from flying out, but to keep owls and hawks from coming in!

7. Half-a-pound of poultry staples to tack top down.

CONSTRUCTION

The selection of the site for the yard is important. It should be on fairly high ground, which is not muddy after every rain. Water birds do like water, but a soggy pen quickly brings parasites and disease. If there is no high ground to use, it would be a very good idea to have a few yards of coarse sand dumped on the highest area available, giving the yard a raised base and good drainage.

The fence posts should be at least a foot-and-a-half or two feet in the ground; otherwise, they will just tip over. If you are not using the two by four-inch braces on the top, the posts must be set at least two-and-a-half feet in the ground. Be sure the posts are straight and are tamped firmly in the ground.

Then, add the two by four-inch top braces. These will prevent the posts from leaning as the wire is pulled tight. They should be nailed on the outside of the pen, with four-inch ringed pole barn nails. These will not pull out. Keep a level handy to be sure the posts do not shift as the braces are nailed in place. A nice square pen is no harder to build than a shabby old one, and it'll make you feel better to look at the nice one. Remember, it will be there for awhile!

After the framework is there, dig a six-inch trench around the base of the yard. This is where the wire will be placed and buried, to prevent any stray animals from digging into your yard. It does happen.

You will need a gate, so add it next. The gate does not have to be wide. We like about a two-foot-wide gate, high enough to walk through comfortably. Make both framework and gate; then add the wire to the gate before hanging it. Then, you can add the wire to the sides of the yard, being very careful to get it tightly stretched and even.

After all of the two by four-inch wire has been stapled down, fill up the trench at the bottom and pack down the dirt well.

The netting top of the yard goes on last. If the yard is large, you may need to add a couple of long poles every 10 feet or so to keep the wire from sagging badly.

If the yard is very large, you may also need to lace two or more widths of netting together to make the top wide enough. Either the netting must be laced together with wire or the edges *must* meet at a pole and both be stapled to it. If there are any gaps in the top, not only might captive birds escape or get injured, but predators may enter and kill the birds.

When the entire yard seems finished, go over your job with a fine-toothed comb, looking for any gaps in the wire, holes under the wire, or unstapled sections. This extra time will really pay off!

If at all possible, give the birds a large pool to bathe and swim in. This can be a children's plastic wading pool, or a more elaborate cement pond. Be sure that the birds can get in *and* out of the pool. If necessary, add large stones for steps, or an easily climbed ramp.

Be sure to change this water as soon as it begins to get foul, as dirty ponds are ideal breeding spots for bacteria, and often cause botulism in water birds. Try to arrange good draining. If possible, syphon the water out of the pool with a garden hose, and into the garden or flower bed. This dirty water is terrific organic fertilizer, but should not just be dumped out in the birds' yard. This will make their yard damp and cause illness or encourage parasite infection.

The birds will need a small shed for protection against the sun and bad weather. If the birds will be wintered over in a cold weather area, this shed will need to be larger. A simple storm shelter needs to be only a little bigger than the birds housed in it, and it can be a three-sided shed, open to the south. However, the winter shed must be larger, preferably at least six feet high (for ease of working in the shed) and large enough to allow the birds some exercise. If the shed is too small, the floor will be constantly wet, no matter how often the bedding is renewed. A large winter shelter is best built outside the birds' yard, with a door providing access to the yard. The door should be constructed so that it can be shut tightly in very bad weather or left open in milder weather.

The winter shelter should not have a pool, or severe dampness will be a problem. To prevent the birds from trying to bathe in their water container, you can fence off a corner with two by four-inch welded wire (unless you are housing very large birds) and place the water container in the corner. The birds can easily reach through the wire to drink, but cannot bathe or splash!

Only in very, very cold climates will heat be needed in a bird shed. And then, only a heat lamp is necessary, provided that the shed is fairly tightly constructed and not too large. In using a heat lamp, *please use extreme caution.* Chain the lamp to the ceiling and protect both lamp and cord from curious birds. Many farm fires have been caused by accidents involving heat lamps.

Feed: Sources, Economics, and Quality

MILK

IN FEEDING ANIMALS, especially baby animals, milk is a common necessity. We have tried just about every type of milk and milk replacer on the market many times—everything from whole, pasteurized milk from the grocery store to powdered, soy flour products.

We believe that the best milk for all baby animals is whole, raw goat milk, mainly because it is very easily digested. The fat globules in goat milk are smaller than in most other milk, giving a lot more surface for digestive processes to act on.

Goat milk is usually easy to get, *but* not all goat milk is good milk. It must come from reasonably healthy goats and be handled in a sanitary manner. Generally, one can decide if the milk is good or not just by taking a quick look at a goat dairy, which may have from 2 to 200 does. If the place is reasonably clean, the goats are clean, and the milk equipment and room are clean, the milk is usually good.

When buying any kind of milk, it is always cheaper to buy it from a producer instead of a local store. When raising any of the smaller animal babies, such as a squirrel, the cost of the milk is not that big an issue. But when you are raising a foal or a moose calf, the milk bill can get awfully big if you are not careful!

It is best not to buy more than five days' milk supply at one time, as the milk should be quite fresh. Remember that raw milk often sours faster than pasteurized milk, as it may contain bacteria which multiply as the days pass, even if the milk is kept below 40°F.

Always be sure to stir up the cream in unhomogenized milk before each use. This is essential to prevent digestive upsets.

If absolutely no cow or goat milk is available and large amounts of milk are needed, you can use a dry calf of lamb milk replacer. Do be sure to get one high in fat and composed of dairy products, such as skim milk, whey, and buttermilk. Such a milk replacer is apt to be higher in price than flour-based replacers, but it is worth the difference in price. Few calves or other animal babies do much, if anything, on cheaper replacers. Try to stay away from medicated milk replacers. Supposedly, the medication is added to help prevent diarrhea, but we have never seen it prevent anything. Moreover, the baby gets so used to the antibiotic in that replacer that even massive dosages of it do little good against diarrhea, pneumonia, or anything else, if the baby should be afflicted. Small babies do well on puppy or kitten formula.

You can locate sources of raw farm milk by simply going from farm to farm and asking if they will sell you raw milk. Dairy goat clubs are also very good in helping to find sources of good quality goat milk.

MEAT

If you are raising any kind of carnivorous baby, sooner or later you will need a good source of meat. And at the prices of meat over the counter, few people can afford to buy enough for the family, let alone for a pet! But there are places where meat for pets can be had, and reasonably too.

First of all, you need to know what kind of meat you will accept. *Never* bring home meat scraps that contain many sharp bone slivers! These sharp pieces will shred the animal's stomach just as they do your fingers.

Your baby can be fed cuts that are not generally used for human consumption. These include clean tripe (stomach lining), hocks, damaged livers, hearts, brains, chicken necks, gizzards, and the like.

Often a rural locker plant or other slaughtering establishment will give you these meat by-products or sell them to you by the pound, along with meat scraps, at a very low price.

Some meat markets will also give or sell, at low prices, boxes of meat scraps and old cuts. Sometimes people will not buy darkened meat, which is perfectly good, and it is thrown into a reject box—or perhaps no one is buying gizzards this week. Ask around. You may have to put up with a lot of quizzical looks and curt answers, but when you do find a free or cheap meat source, you will have found a gold mine. Hang on to it. Always be on time, be polite, and show a respect for the rules of the business.

When you are feeding a bird of prey or other baby that needs bone and hair, the slaughterhouse can provide you with that too. Remember, though, that most scraps and bones should not be fed cooked, but raw. When bones are cooked, they become brittle, splinter easily, and often kill animals by puncturing the digestive tract or becoming jammed in the intestines so badly that they completely block them. Death quickly results. Birds of prey can also be fed pet shop or trapped mice and other wild rodents.

Do not accept any rancid or spoiled meat or meat scraps—or if you do, deposit them immediately in the garbage can. Don't keep them or try to use them as feed. Some animals can eat spoiled meat just fine. But it can kill. Give all your meat the "sniff" test, just to be sure!

BREAD

Bread is needed in large amounts when many different babies are being raised at once or a large baby, such as a bear, is being fed. A large bear can go through several loaves of bread a day with ease! And that translates into a lot of money, especially when added to the other food consumed daily.

We have found that the largest supplies of bread are found at the big commercial bakeries. When you only need a few loaves a week for your babies, that small, local, home-owned bakery down the street will do fine, but when you need volume, go commercial.

Commercial bakeries generally place bread in stores daily, or every other day, and take all baked goods that are not sold back to their home outlet. Here they are sold by the pound, sometimes given away or even thrown out. Often, you can purchase 50 pounds of bread for the cost of three loaves in your local grocery store.

This bread is often a bit smashed up, sometimes a bit stale, and once in awhile a little moldy. But, for the most part, it is quite good animal food. We prefer to stay away from bread containing many preservatives. If you shop well (and you should, even for your animal babies), you can find low-preservative content in bargain basement bread.

You can find such bakery outlets by asking your local stores who supplies them, and then make a few person-to-person visits. Phone calls usually net only negative replies. Be sure you ask for bread for animal food, not day-old bread. The day-old bread costs much more and is often the same bread that is sold for "animal food." Do not feed bread that is very moldy. A small bit of bread mold will do no harm, but large amounts of mold can cause digestive problems. Do not let the animal have the bread in plastic wraps. Often the animals will eat some of the plastic, causing intestinal blockages and death.

DOG AND CAT FOOD

When you keep only a pet dog or cat, feeding is fairly inexpensive. But, when you are raising a litter of medium to large-size breed puppies, or are feeding a kennel of dogs or many cats, you can quickly learn to feel panic during every trip to the store!

As a whole, canned foods are out. True, dogs and cats like them better than their dry counterparts, but canned food costs more and is often less nutritious. We use canned foods as a treat (often mixed with dry food) or to tempt a pup, kitten, or sick animal to eat.

With these foods you should be especially careful to read labels. Often a food will sound good, have a pretty label, be reasonably priced, and be composed of junk! Now, by junk we mean such things as hair, ground bones, and feathers. Don't laugh. Some unscrupulous feed dealers use these things to boost the protein content of the food. Don't automatically assume it is nutritious just because a food contains 24% protein. *Read the label.* You should find that the food contains: meat by-products, cottage cheese, dried whey, soybean oil meal, and other good nutrients.

When a label reads: ground cereal grains, dried brewer's grains, fish by-products, and a list of vitamins (or some such), it contains more of the first ingredient than the next, and on down the line. And ground cereal grains are not a good primary ingredient for a carnivore. It is best to stay with the better known dog and cat food companies. This food usually costs a bit more but, in general, the ingredients are researched for food value, and the quality is maintained.

To offset the cost of the food, write to the companies and ask if they have a group or breeder discount or club. They usually do, which means that you get a rebate or discount when you buy. This can add up to quite a saving for someone who uses a lot of feed!

You also might check with your grocery or feed dealer to see if he or she will cut the price to you if you buy a large amount at one time. We have had quite good luck with this, but have had to buy a ton of dog food at a time, or 500 pounds of cat food. If you have good, vermin- and rodent-free storage areas and will use the food within a month or two, this can be a very economical way to buy. But, don't allow the food to become damp or damaged by rodents and insects. Also, don't keep feed too long, as you will often lose nutrients as the food becomes stale and the fats get rancid.

Most times cats do well on a dry diet, but there are a few cautions. Cats can get cystitis (infection or blockage of the urinary tract) from eating a dry diet. This is thought to be because they do not get enough water, unlike when a canned food is fed (canned foods are often 70 percent water). This is most often seen in males, particularly altered males. Should this condition be a worry, or if it has happened, canned foods may be necessary. In some areas cystitis is seldom seen, regardless of diet; in others it is very common. Ask cat owners and veterinarians. If yours seems to be a "high risk" area, it would be best to feed a canned food.

But not all canned food is good canned food! Remember: first read the label; if cystitis is a problem, feed a low-ash and low-fish diet (a meat- or poultry-based food is best). Be careful. Even beef-liver *flavored* cat food is often made up with a fish by-product base!

Frequently, canned foods can be bought from your grocer or feed dealer by the case, at a considerable saving. In general larger cans are more economical than those little single-serving cans. But, don't be fooled into substituting quantity for quality!

After canned foods are opened, cover them with plastic to avoid their drying out between feedings, and refrigerate the leftovers. Not only are dry leftovers that have been left out on the counter all day unappetizing, but they can contain very deadly bacteria.

HAY AND STRAW

Hay is well-dried grass or legumes (clover, alfalfa, or vetch) that (hopefully) has been cut before it got mature and tough. Straw is the fully mature leftover stalk from cereal grains (wheat, oats, barley, or rye). Straw is yellow, hollow, fully mature, and very low in feed value. It is usually used for bedding, where hay is used for feed.

As in many cases, both hay and straw are cheapest when they are bought directly from the farmer, cutting out many middlemen. We have seen tiny bags of hay offered in pet shops for three times what a whole bale of hay sells for at a farm! But then there is a feed dealer, a trucker, a packaging plant, wholesaler, another trucker, and pet shop all making a living from that tiny bag!

For general use, a good mixed hay is best. A mixed hay usually contains both grasses and a legume. An example would be orchard grass and timothy mixed with red clover. A pure legume hay, such as alfalfa, is often very high in protein, but also tends to loosen the bowels and to cause digestive upsets. A pure grass hay is lower in protein and is not relished as much as the legume or legume-mixed hay.

Any hay should be bright green, dust-free, and smell *terrific.* Hay should not be yellowish on the outside, have black spots, or have a blue dust (mold) when the bale is opened. Not only do animals dislike dusty or moldy hay, but it can cause severe digestive upsets, respiratory trouble, and can even poison the animal. Moldy sweet clover (not usually found in hay) produces a deadly poison.

Hay and straw can either be bought by the bale or by the ton. Buying by the ton is better, when possible. The size of the bale can be regulated when the hay is baled, and a few farmers make very short, light bales, when they know they will be selling hay! A bale of hay can weigh anywhere from 20 pounds to over 90 pounds, so when hay is priced by the bale, you must be a good judge of weight to estimate the true worth of your "buy."

Generally, wire-tied bales are the heaviest, and small round bales the lightest and hardest to load, stack, and handle.

Both hay and straw must be stored inside, or be well-protected outdoors. When it is rained on, the water seeps deep into the pile, quickly causing the nice pile of hay or straw to become a hot pile of compost. Even when hay is piled on the ground, inside a building, it should be elevated on a layer of old car tires to keep the bales from absorbing ground water or dampness, which rots the bottom layer.

PASTURE

All of the grasses and legumes grown for hay can be used for a pasture. There are two basic types of pasture: wild and planted. A wild pasture is one that is made up of native grasses that have not been planted by man. This type of pasture is fine in many areas, but it does have the disadvantage of becoming sod-bound after several years, which severely decreases the amount of forage available within a set area.

In most cases, it is much more economical to have a pasture renewed every few years. Renewal consists of having the pasture, all or half of it, plowed up, fertilized, and limed where needed (have a soil sample checked to be sure), then harrowed and smoothed and finally seeded. Just sowing seed in an unworked pasture may net you some new plants, but the sod-bound condition will still exist, and the plants will not do much.

Your county agent will be of great assistance in helping you to determine which grasses and legumes to use, and he can help you learn to take a soil sample. He will probably recommend a commercial fertilizer, but good old barnyard manure will do just fine. Do heed his recommendations to add lime to the soil, if needed. It will really boost the pasture!

It is usually best to plant a mixed pasture, as a straight legume pasture can cause digestive upsets like colic, founder, bloat, and diarrhea. A pasture is usually planted in the spring, using one of the grains, such as oats for a nurse crop. The nurse crop is planted somewhat lighter than if it were being planted strictly for grain. This nurse crop helps protect the new seeding from wind, sun, and rain. The grain is cut at maturity, giving grain, straw, and a new seeding from one field. It is best not to pasture the new pasture at all, but if it is badly needed, it can receive light grazing in the fall. *Never* turn animals into a new seeding in wet weather. Their feet will churn the tender new plants into the ground and leave bad ruts and holes for years to come.

Never turn animals used to hay only onto a lush pasture. They will overeat and can even die. It is much better to gradually introduce them to the pasture, grazing them for only an hour at first, and slowly increasing their time out on the grass.

GRAIN

Grain is the backbone in feeding many animals. In ruminants, grain provides the needed protein and extra carbohydrates, while hay and pasture provide the bulk and roughage. Ruminants need the roughage to keep their rumen working. Where only grain or large amounts of grain are fed, the rumen becomes acid, killing off vital bacteria. Soon the animal is off feed, and it can be very hard to get it back to normal again.

Few animals do well on one grain alone. True, when you think of horses, you think of oats. But, oats is not enough for a horse that is growing, is used for breeding, or is working hard. Pigs bring to mind corn. But, corn alone will not support growth or breeding activity. It is only to fatten pigs. Most animals do best on a mixed grain ration, as do humans.

The grains used depend a lot on the area, but generally, oats, corn, and soybean-oil meal are in many rations. These ingredients balance and support each other. Unless you intend to do a lot of study on balancing a ration, it is best to use a mixed grain, formulated by a local feed mill. These mixed rations are usually quite stable in ingredients and nutrients. *Be sure to read the label, or find out for sure what is in the mix.* If in doubt, take the label to your veterinarian or county agent.

It is generally cheaper to buy grain by the ton, rather than buy it in those nice, heavy paper bags holding only 50 pounds. We save over $50 by buying by the ton, compared with buying the 50-pound sack. The only problem with buying by the ton is the need for good storage facilities. If you are going to use a lot of grain, there is seldom any problem. But, when only a few animals are fed, the grain can become stale and contaminated by rodents and insects. The grain bin must be weather-tight and dry. If a ton of grain cannot be fed up within a month and a half, you'd better buy your grain by the 100-pound sack. This is still cheaper than the paper sacks in most cases, and more economical than having part of the ton go to waste or become spoiled.

A large metal garbage can with a lid makes a good feed bin for 100 pounds of grain. Be sure that the grain is stored away from the animals. They can knock over the can, flip off the lid, and eat a lot of grain in no time. Not only does this waste grain, but it can kill the animals too.

PELLETS

Many types of animal feed are pelletized. In this process, the feed is ground fine, then pressed through a pelletizing machine under high pressure. The pellets are quite dust-free, and they do not allow the animal to sort through the feed, only eating the parts it likes best. Rabbits, cavies (guinea pigs), dogs, horses, goats, sheep, pigs, calves, cows, monkeys, and birds all have some pelletized feed available.

Some of the pelletized feed is a complete food. The best example of this is rabbit pellets. This is fine in some cases, making feeding very timesaving. But some animals, such as horses, eat the pellets quickly and still have the urge to eat more so they begin chewing at their stall or fences. Should this occur, add some grass hay to the diet.

Be very sure of the contents of the pellets! Read the label very carefully. We have seen a lot of cheaper pellets with poor nutrients. If in doubt, again, take the label to your veterinarian or county agent.

BIRD SEED

As with other feeds, when you buy bird seed, it is not always cheaper to buy inexpensive seed. Some cheaper seed, often sold at grocery stores and cut-rate stores, is not digestible or even palatable to birds. But it is cheap to grow and makes a cheap filler for bags of seed.

Good quality seed can often be bought reasonably in bulk from a feed dealer or a pet shop. This is especially true of sunflower seed and millet.

It is a good idea to contact a local bird fancier, whether the person raises birds or just feeds wild birds. This person can advise you on

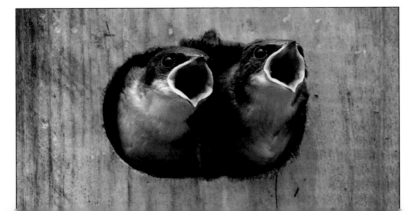

what types of seeds you should look for, and the types preferred by birds in your neighborhood. He or she can also tell you the most economical place to buy good seed.

Be absolutely sure that the seed is stored away from rodents and dampness. A clean metal garbage can makes an ideal storage container for large amounts of seed.

TABLE SCRAPS

Table scraps can be the best food additive for your animals—or the worst. The difference depends on a few things. First, you must consider the quality of the table scraps for the animal you are going to feed. Some animals can tolerate all household garbage, and make good use of it. The two at the top of this list are chickens and hogs. But, even these animals must be fed fresh, uncontaminated garbage! All sorts of kitchen by-products can be added to the diet of a flock of chickens or a pig, from wholesome, but soured milk to potato peelings. Ours get all the juice from canned goods, vegetable scraps, dry bread crusts, leftovers, and such.

But, all animals cannot be fed all scraps. The house dog and cat are two of the ones that often suffer from the wrong table scraps. *Never* give them cooked, small bones. Chicken bones, pork bones, steak bones, and fish bones are often fed, and they often kill the animals! Many people say, "We've fed Spot bones all his life, and they never hurt him." But we see many animals each month that *were* hurt by those well-meant bones.

A dog might like some foods that are not necessarily good for it. For instance, highly spiced foods, fried foods and high-starch foods can cause indigestion. This is not to say that a dog cannot have a few fat scraps or leftover taco now and then. But a small dog cannot be fed a *lot* of this type food, or most of its diet will turn out to be undesirable foods, and it may be in trouble quickly.

Be sure that the animal will get a good *balanced* diet, and that the table scraps are only "goodies" or additions to the diet.

We see an awful lot of very overweight dogs and cats—who get an abundance of table scraps, and will "not touch" dry foods. They are spoiled by well-meaning people and usually have health troubles because of it.

FRUITS AND VEGETABLES

Fruits and vegetables can make up a sizable portion of the diet for many animals. A home garden and orchard are ideal sources for adding these things to your animal's diet. There are many rejects and by-products from the garden that are relished by animals. These may be: tomatoes with spots, overripe produce, small or misshapen fruits and vegetables, peelings, and pieces left over at canning time, leaves and vines, sweet corncobs, thinned vegetables, windfall fruit, and so on. Many people even plant extra vegetables, just for their animals.

You might want to contact local fruit and vegetable stands to see if they have leftover produce that is unsalable, but still fit for animals to eat. Grocery stores also can be of help. They often have boxes of vegetable trimmings and assorted throw-away produce. A word of caution: please wash the produce well, as much commercially grown produce is loaded with insecticides!

SPECIAL DIETS

There are many specialized diets available today. Most of these are a bit costly, but are downright convenient and highly nutritious. They are also much easier to use than concocting a balanced diet every day!

There are special diets for monkeys, carnivorous birds, fruit eaters, dogs with intestinal or kidney problems, puppies, deer, game birds, pigeons, and so on. You can find out more about these diets by contacting your local veterinarian, pet shop, or zoo.

EGGS

Hard-boiled eggs and hard-boiled and mashed egg yolks are often a good first solid food for baby birds and animals. But there is no need to spend what it costs for a dozen grade-A eggs at the grocery store. A short trip into the country will usually net you a very cheap (sometimes free) source of eggs!

Many commercial egg houses, which may have over 12,000 hens in just one chicken house, usually have many eggs that they don't sell to wholesalers or private people. These are actually those eggs that have a blood spot. A small blood spot on the yolk is completely harmless and is simply caused by a tiny ruptured blood vessel in the hen's oviduct. But it does not look "nice" on a breakfast plate. This is the primary reason that eggs are candled in commercial egg "factories." These blood-spotted eggs are often given away for animal food—or even thrown out! Those blood spots don't bother animals one bit. There are also pullet eggs, which are smaller and therefore cheaper.

Eggs are best fed boiled, poached, or baked. Fried eggs are not good for any animal. When many eggs are to be fed, the quickest method is to bake them. This does away with the tedious job of shelling boiled eggs. Simply separate yolk from white, if desired, slip the yolk into a pan, then repeat until enough eggs are ready. Then, simply pop the pan into the oven at 300°F until the eggs are done.

Another possible source of eggs for animal food is a hatchery. Here you may be able to pick up eggs that are not fertile. Unless they are old, they will be fine for your animal and bird babies. Sniff each egg as you open it, however. If one is spoiled, you will quickly notice that fact!

If you are really concerned with the diet of your babies, read all you can about them. One good, all-around book on feeding, which shows just what is in just about every food available, is *Feeds and Feeding* by Arthur E. Cullison (2d ed., Reston, Virginia: Reston Publishing Co., 1979.) This book is available at most public libraries.

First Aid Equipment to Have on Hand

HORSES		(F = FOAL, A = ADULT)
Thermometer	to check temperature rectally	f and a
Scissors	for clipping hair away from wounds, cutting bandages, etc.	f and a
Syringe, 12 cc. Needle, 18 gauge 1 inch	for giving intramuscular (IM), subcutaneous (SC) injections	f and a
Balling gun:	for giving boluses	
calf size		f
regular size		a
Cotton	for wrapping legs, packing wounds, and cleaning	f and a
Ace bandage or horse-leg wrap	for wrapping legs, keeping pressure on wounds, and shipping protection	f and a
Iodine	for treating small cuts and dipping foal's navel (at birth)	f and a
Antibiotic or sulfa powder	to "puff" onto wounds	f and a
Pen-strep (Combiotic)	100 cc for treating many infections and illnesses	f and a
Kaolin-pectin	basic diarrhea medication	f
Oral electrolytes	used in treating diarrhea	f
Lamb nipple and quart pop bottle	for feeding orphan foal	f
Feeding tube 22 inch French size 12 or 14	for feeding weak foal	f
Old intravenous (IV) outfit, less needle and hub	to attach to above feeding tube and to bottle of milk for tube-feeding weak foal	f

CATTLE		(C = CALF, A = ADULT)
Thermometer	to check temperature rectally	c and a
Scissors	for clipping hair away from wounds, cutting bandages, etc.	c and a
Syringe, 12 cc. Needle, 18 gauge 1 inch	for giving intramuscular (IM), subcutaneous (SC) injections	c and a
Needle, 18 gauge 3 inch	for giving interperitoneal (IP) injections	c and a
Intravenous (IV) outfit	for giving weak or dehydrated calf IP injections	c
Balling gun:	for giving boluses	
calf size		c
regular size		a
Cotton	for packing wounds and cleaning	c and a
Antibiotic or sulfa powder	to "puff" onto wounds	c and a
Iodine	for treating small cuts and dipping calf's navel (at birth)	c and a
Udder ointment	for treating mastitis, chapped teats, and chapped nose (calf)	c and a
Eye powder	for treating pinkeye and other eye injuries and infections	c and a
Louse powder	for eliminating lice in winter (use once monthly)	c and a
Penicillin or other injectable antibiotic. (Combiotic)	100 cc for treating many infections, pneumonia, and mastitis (milk from cattle being treated with this drug *must* be withheld from market for at least 96 hours after last injection)	c and a

Kaolin-pectin	basic diarrhea medication	c
Oral electrolytes	used in treating diarrhea	c
Injectable electrolytes	used in treating severe diarrhea and also dehydration in fever	c
Calf bottle	for feeding young calf	c
Feeding tube 22 inch French size 14	for feeding weak calf	c
Old IV outfit, less needle and hub	to attach to above feeding tube and to bottle of milk for tube-feeding weak calf	c
SWINE		**(P = PIGLET, A = ADULT)**
Thermometer	to check temperature rectally	p and a
Scissors	for clipping hair away from wounds, trimming newborn pig's unbilical cord, cutting bandages, etc.	p and a
Side-cutters	to clip new pig's needle teeth and clip tail, if desired	p
Syringes:	for giving intramuscular (IM), subcutaneous (SC) injections	
6 cc.		p
12 cc.		a
Needles: 20 gauge 1 inch	for giving intramuscular (IM), subcutaneous (SC) injections	p
18 gauge 1 inch		a
Iodine	for treating small cuts, docked tails, and dipping piglet's navel (at birth)	p and a
Antibiotic or sulfa powder	to "puff" onto wounds	p and a

Penicillin or other injectable antibiotic. (Combiotic)	for treating many infections, pneumonia, etc.	p and a
Kaolin-pectin	basic diarrhea medication	p
Oral electrolytes	used in treating diarrhea	p and a
Injectable iron	to prevent anemia in babies	p
Human baby bottle	for feeding very young baby pig	p
Feeding tube 16 inch French size 8 or 10	for feeding weak piglet	p
SHEEP AND GOATS		**(K OR l = KID OR LAMB, A = ADULT)**
Thermometer	to check temperature rectally	k, l, and a
Scissors	for clipping hair or wool away from wounds, trimming loose flaps of skin away from wounds, cutting bandages, etc.	k, l, and a
Syringes:	for giving intramuscular (IM), subcutaneous (SC) injections	
6 cc.		k and l
12 cc.		a
Needles: 20 gauge 1 inch	for giving intramuscular (IM), subcutaneous (SC) injections	k and l
18 gauge 1 inch		a
Needles: 18 gauge 2 inch	for giving interperitoneal (IP) injections	k and l
16 gauge 2 inch		a
Intravenous (IV) outfit	for giving IP injections for weakness or dehydration	k, l, and a

Balling gun, calf size	for giving boluses	a
Liquid Ivory (or similar dish soap)	lubrication for hands when aiding a difficult birth	a
Iodine	for treating small cuts, ringworm, and dipping newborn's navel	k, l, and a
Udder ointment	for treating chapped or scratched teats, congested udder, or soreness from mastitis	a
Scarlet oil	used on wounds during fly season to prevent maggots and to aid healing	k, l, and a
Antibiotic or sulfa powder	to "puff" onto wounds	k, l, and a
Eye powder	for treating pinkeye and other eye injuries and infections	k, l, and a
Penicillin or other injectable antibiotic. (Combiotic)	for treating many infections, pneumonia, and mastitis (milk from animals being treated with this drug *must* be withheld from market for at least 96 hours after last injection)	k, l, and a
Kaolin-pectin	basic diarrhea medication	k, l, and a
Subnet (sulfamethazine)	given orally to prevent and treat infections and coccidiosis	k, l, and a
Oral electrolytes	used in treating diarrhea	k, l, and a
Injectable electrolytes	used in treating severe diarrhea and also dehydration in fever	k, l, and a
Clean, used 12-cc. syringe	for giving liquid orally	k and l
Lamb nipple and quart pop bottle	for feeding babies	k and l
Feeding tube 16 inch French size 8 or 10	for feeding weak babies	k and l

SMALLER ANIMALS (DOGS, CATS, WILD DOGS, WILD CATS, RODENTS, RACCOONS, OPOSSUMS, AND THE LIKE)		(B = BABY, A = ADULT)
Thermometer	to check temperature rectally	b and a
Scissors	for clipping hair away from wounds, cutting bandages, etc.	b and a
Syringe, 6 cc. Needle, 20 gauge 1 inch	for giving intramuscular (IM), subcutaneous (SC) injections	b and a
Cotton	for packing wounds and cleaning	b and a
Gauze bandage (1 inch, in rolls)	to wrap bleeding wounds	b and a
Triple sulfa tablets	to treat many infections	b and a
Antibiotic or sulfa powder	used to "puff" onto wounds	b and a
Penicillin or other injectable antibiotic. (Combiotic)	for treating many infections, pneumonia, etc.	b and a
Kaolin-pectin	basic diarrhea medication	b and a
Subnet (sulfamethazine)	given orally to prevent and treat infections and coccidiosis	b and a
Oral electrolytes	used in treating diarrhea	b and a
Injectable electrolytes	used in treating diarrhea and also dehydration in fever	b and a
Clean, used 6-cc. syringe	for giving liquid orally	b and a
Pet nurser	for feeding most babies	b
Feeding tube 16-inch French size 3 to 8	for feeding weak babies	b
Syringe, 12 cc.	for tube-feeding	b

BIRDS		(B = BABY, A = ADULT)
Scissors	for clipping small, loose flaps of skin away from wounds, cutting bandages, etc.	b and a
Tweezers	for removing feathers, gravel, etc., from injured area	b and a
Cotton	for packing wounds, cleaning, and as nest for small babies	b and a
Gauze bandage (1 inch, in rolls)	to wrap injuries and immobilize injured wings	b and a
Styptic powder	for minor bleeding, as often seen in torn nails	b and a
Eye ointment	for treating eye injuries and infections	b and a
Bonemeal	needed especially by birds of prey	b and a
Sulmet (sulfamethazine)	given orally to prevent and treat infections and coccidiosis	b and a
Oral electrolytes	used in treating dehydration, especially in waterfowl	a
Multiple vitamin drops (infant)	very helpful in preventing vitamin deficiencies in hand-raised birds	b
Small, blunt sticks	to help feed babies, acting as "beak" of mother, holding food	b

Body Temperature Chart

AS STATED MANY, many times throughout this book, body temperature is a very important clue to the state of an animal's health. A raised temperature often indicates a bacterial infection, a virus, or possible overheating. A lowered temperature can point to internal bleeding, shock, severe chill, or even the imminent death of the animal.

When an animal acts a little "off," take its temperature first of all—*before giving that shot, before calling the vet, and before putting it in a warm place!*

The "normal" temperatures, listed below are just that. A few animals carry a naturally higher (slightly) temperature than the "normal," but if it is quite a bit higher, or lower, than the normal, you can bet something is wrong—especially if the animal has been acting depressed in the first place.

NORMAL TEMPERATURE RANGES
(ALL TEMPERATURES, TAKEN RECTALLY, ARE GIVEN IN DEGREES FAHRENHEIT.)

Mouse	97-97.5	Small monkey	102.5-103.5
Rat	100.2-101	Sheep	102-102.5
Chipmunk	98.6-99	Goat	101.5-102.5
Rabbit	102-102.5	Pig	101-102
Raccoon	102-102.5	Deer	101.5-102.5
Cat	101.5-101.8	Cow	101.5-102
Dog	101.5-102	Donkey	100.5-101
Bobcat	101-101.5	Horse	100-100.5

Glossary

Abdominal cavity: the part of the body containing organs, such as stomach, kidneys, liver, spleen, uterus (female) and intestines

Abortion: the termination of a pregnancy before term

Afterbirth: the placenta which is expelled during or after the birth of a mammal

Anemia: a condition in which the blood is deficient in red blood cells, hemoglobin, or volume

Antibiotic: a substance which inhibits or kills bacterial organisms

Aspiration pneumonia: pneumonia caused by inhalation of fluid or dust

Bacteria: one-celled organisms belonging to the plant family

Bonemeal: an inexpensive and easily obtained source of calcium

Botulism: a condition, often called food poisoning, caused by bacterial contamination of food or fouled water

Caesarean section: removal of the fetus through an incision in the abdominal wall

Coccidiosis: infestation by a parasitic protozoa, characterized by diarrhea, stunted growth, and unthriftiness; often treated with sulfas

Concussion: an injury to the brain, caused by a fall or blow

Constipation: an inability to defecate, often due to starvation, fever, or illness

Dehydration: serious loss of body salts, chemicals, and fluids

De-scenting: removal of the scent glands. Goats (bucks only) on head; ferrets and skunks, next to rectum

Diarrhea: fluid texture of stools, often copiously discharged

Distemper: a contagious, often fatal disease, found in many animals; symptoms often include: fever, discharge from eyes and nose

Electrolytes: normal bases, acids, and salts found in the blood

Expectorant: a substance which clears the air passages of secretions

Farrow: to give birth to pigs; also a litter of pigs

Fecal: pertaining to bowel movements

Feline distemper: see Panleucopenia

Fetus: an unborn, developing animal

French feeding tube: a flexible tube used to deposit milk into the stomach directly, without the baby animal's sucking

Frostbite: the freezing of some part of the body, such as the ears; characterized by stiffness, swelling and whiteness in the area (later redness)

Grub: a wormlike form of insect larva

Hand-raise: to raise a baby animal without benefit of a mother or nurse

Hemorrhage: heavy or uncontrollable bleeding

Impaction: a blockage of the bowel

Intramedullary pin: a stainless steel pin which goes in the marrow cavity; used to repair broken bones

Intramuscular (IM) injection: injection given deep into a muscle

Intraperitoneal (IP) injection: injection given into the abdominal cavity

Joint ill: infection of a joint, often caused by not dipping the navel in iodine at birth

Kaolin-pectin: a thick, chalky substance given to treat diarrhea

Mange: a condition of the skin, caused by tiny mites; symptoms include itching, red skin, and scabs

Ophthalmic: pertaining to the eye

Overeating disease (enterotoxemia): a disease which can be prevented by vaccination; causes sudden death, diarrhea, uncoordination, and weakness in sheep, calves, and goats

Panleucopenia: a very contagious, quick-striking, often fatal disease of cats, raccoons, ferrets, coatimundis, and some other wild animals; characterized by diarrhea, vomiting, depression and often, quick death

Parasite: an organism living in or on another, depending on its host for support and/or existence

Placenta: the organ in which the fetus is wrapped before birth; expelled during or after birth

Rotenone: a plant-derived, quite safe insecticide

Ruminants: animals that chew a cud, such as deer, cattle, goats, and sheep

Scours: severe diarrhea in animals

Subcutaneous (SC) injection: an injection given just under the skin

Suture: to sew (as in a wound); also a threadlike material used to sew

Syringe: an instrument used to inject fluid into, or remove fluid from, the body

Tetanus: an acute, often fatal disease, caused by an organism, often introduced into the body through a wound; characterized by stiffness, inability to eat and appearance of white membrane from corner of eye

Tube-feeding: see French feeding tube

Tuberculosis (TB): a contagious disease in animals and man, usually involving the lungs

Umbilical: pertaining to the depressed area in the center of the abdomen; the navel

Vaccine: a suspension of live, killed, or weakened virus or bacteria, administered to the body to build up immunity to diseases caused by those organisms

Virus: a microorganism that reproduces itself and obtains energy from the body cells it enters, causing damage to the cells from within

Wean: to remove bottle-fed or other forms of sole milk diet from an infant animal

HERE ARE SOME SOURCES OF BABY ANIMAL SUPPLIES:

DRS. FOSTER AND SMITH

1-800-381-7179

HOEGGER SUPPLY COMPANY

1-800-221-4628

JEFFERS PET SUPPLY

1-800-533-3377

KV SUPPLY

1-800-423-8211

NASCO FARM AND RANCH

1-800-558-9595

VALLEY VET SUPPLY

1-800-419-9524

Suggested Reading

WILD ANIMALS

Adamson, Joy. *Born Free.* New York: Random House, 1974.

——. *Forever Free.* New York: Harcourt Brace Jovanovich, 1963.

——. *Living Free.* New York: Harcourt Brace Jovanovich, 1961.

——. *Pippa's Challenge.* New York: Harcourt Brace Jovanovich, 1972.

——. *The Spotted Sphinx.* New York: Harcourt Brace Jovanovich, 1969.

Ms. Adamson's books are rich in enchanting stories of the joy and pain that come of close personal contact with wild babies in raising them for release.

Austing, G. Ronald. *The World of the Red-Tailed Hawk.* Living World Books Series. Philadelphia: J. B. Lippincott Co., 1964.

Austing, G. Ronald, and Holt, John B. Jr. *The World of the Great Horned Owl.* Living World Books Series. Philadelphia: J. B. Lippincott Co., 1966.

Costello, David F. *The World of the Porcupine.* Living World Books Series. Philadelphia: J. B. Lippincott Co., 1966.

Rue, Leonard Lee III. *The World of the Beaver.* Living World Books Series. Philadelphia: J. B. Lippincott Co., 1964.

——. *The World of the Raccoon.* Living World Books Series. Philadelphia: J. B. Lippincott Co., 1964.

——. *The World of the White-Tailed Deer.* Living World Books Series. Philadelphia: J. B. Lippincott Co., 1962.

Van Wormer, Joe. *The World of the Black Bear.* Living World Books Series. Philadelphia: J. B. Lippincott Co., 1967.

——. *The World of the Bobcat.* Living World Books Series. Philadelphia: J. B. Lippincott Co., 1964.

——. *The World of the Coyote.* Living World Books Series. Philadelphia: J. B. Lippincott Co., 1965.

All of the books that comprise the above series are very easy reading, each containing good photography and a lot of information.

Bent, Arthur C. *Life Histories of North American Birds of Prey.* 2 vols. Magnolia, Mass.: Peter Smith Publisher, 1958.

Use this set to get acquainted with each group of birds more closely.

Collett, Rosemary K., and Briggs, Charlie. *Rescue and Home Care of Native Wildlife.* New York: Hawthorn Books, 1976.

This unusual book deals mainly with Southern animals and especially shore and water birds. One of the best on birds that are found in swampy areas.

Crisler, Lois. *Arctic Wild.* New York: Harper & Row Publishers, 1973.

——. *Captive Wild.* New York: Harper & Row Publishers, 1968.

Both books deal specifically with wolves in contact with human beings and are terrific reading.

Grossman, Mary Louise, and Hamlet, John N. *Birds of Prey of the World.* New York: Clarkson N. Potter, 1965.

This is a good aid to identifying birds of prey and learning more about their diet and habits.

Hickman, Mae, and Guy, Maxine. *Care of the Wild Feathered and Furred: A Guide to Wildlife Handling and Care.* Santa Cruz, Calif.: Unity Press, 1973.

We recommend this as a good general book. It contains a good feed chart.

Leslie, Robert Franklin. *The Bears and I.* New York: E. P. Dutton, 1968.

This book is the true story of a man who raised three bears in the North, from cub to adult. It gives a picture of what life is like with three bear "children."

Line, Les, and Russell, Franklin. *Audubon Society Book of Wild Birds.* New York: Harry N. Abrams, 1976.

This classic offers good photos and lots of vital information.

Martini, Helen. *My Zoo Family.* New York: Harper & Row Publishers, 1955.

This book gives numerous examples of personal involvement with
many different types of baby animals.

North, Sterling. *Raccoons Are the Brightest People.* New York: E. P. Dutton, 1966.

——. *Rascal.* New York: Avon Books, 1969.

These are the two best books on raccoons and the raccoon-person
relationship.

Rawlings, Marjorie K. *The Yearling.* Illustrated Classics. New York:
Charles Scribner's Sons, 1962.

Although this book is fiction, it does present a true picture of raising
a fawn.

Rood, Ronald. *The Loon in My Bathtub.* Brattleboro, Vt: Stephen Greene
Press, 1974.

Look here for a lot of personal tips on raising a variety of animal
babies; includes pond life.

Service, William. *Owl.* New York: Alfred A. Knopf, 1969.

Service's biography of an owl gives terrific insight into the bird's
feeding, personality, and habits.

Stanger, Margaret A. *That Quail, Robert.* New York: Fawcett Book
Group, 1978.

Margaret Stanger's book about Robert is much more than just another
"story." The book takes him from egg to household pet and does a
good job all the way through.

DOMESTIC ANIMALS

GOATS

Books

Belanger, Jerome. *Raising Milk Goats the Modern Way.* Charlotte, Vt:
Garden Way Publishing, 1975.

Colby, Byron E. et al. *Dairy Goats—Breeding, Feeding and Management.*
Spindale, N.C.: American Dairy Goat Association, 1972.

Eberhardt, Jo. *Good Beginnings with Dairy Goats.* Scottsdale, Ariz.:
Dairy Goat Journal Publishing Corp., 1975.

Magazine

Dairy Goat Journal, Dairy Goat Journal Publishing Corp., P.O. Box 1908, Scottsdale, AZ 85252.

SHEEP
Books

Bradbury, Margaret. *Shepherd's Guidebook: Raising Sheep for Meat, Wool, and Hides.* Emmaus, Pa.: Rodale Press, 1977.

Juergenson, Elwood M. *Approved Practices in Sheep Production.* Danville, Ill.: Interstate, 1973.

Simmons, Paula. *Raising Sheep the Modern Way.* Charlotte, Vt: Garden Way Publishing, 1975.

Magazine

Shepherd and Sheep Raiser, A. A. Lund Associates, Sheffield, MA 01257.

RABBITS
Books

Bennett, Robert. *Raising Rabbits the Modern Way.* Charlotte, Vt: Garden Way Publishing, 1975.

Kanable, Ann. *Raising Rabbits.* Emmaus, Pa.: Rodale Press, 1977.

Templeton, George S. *Domestic Rabbit Production.* Danville, Ill: Interstate, 1968.

POULTRY AND WATERFOWL
Books

Delacour, Jean. *Pheasant Breeding and Care.* Neptune, N.J.: T. F. H. Publishers, n.d.

Luttmann, Rick, and Luttmann, Gail. *Chickens in Your Backyard.* Emmaus, Pa.: Rodale Press, 1976.

Naether, Carl. *Making Squab Raising Profitable.* Pine River, Minn.: Stromberg Publishing Co., 1973.

Scheid, Dan W. *Raising Game Birds*. Pine River, Minn.: Stromberg Publishing Co., n.d.

Sheraw, Darrel. *Successful Duck and Goose Raising*. Pine River, Minn.: Stromberg Publishing Co., 1976.

Stromberg, Janet. *A Guide to Better Hatching*. Pine River, Minn.: Stromberg Publishing Co., 1974.

Stromberg, Loyl. *Sexing All Fowl, Baby Chicks, Game Birds, Cage Birds*. Pine River, Minn.: Stromberg Publishing Co., 1977.

Van Hoesen and Stromberg. *Guinea Fowl*. Pine River, Minn.: Stromberg Publishing Co., 1976.

Magazines and Newsletters

American Bantam Association, Box 610, N. Amherst, MA 01059. Newsletter.

American Poultry Association, Box 70, Cushing, OK 74023. Newsletter.

Backyard Poultry, Countryside Publishers, Rt. 1, Box 7C, Waterloo, WI 53594.

Game Bird Breeders, Aviculturists, Zoologists, and Conservationists Gazette, Allen Publishing Co., 1155 East 4785 South, Salt Lake City, UT 84117.

Poultry Press, Box 947, York, PA 17405.

CATTLE

Books

Grohman, Merril, and Grohman, Joann. *The Cow Economy*. Dixfield, Maine: Coburn Farm Press, 1975.

Hobson, Phyllis. *Raising A Calf for Beef*. Charlotte, Vt: Garden Way Publishing, 1976.

Van Loon, Dirk. *The Family Cow*. Charlotte, Vt: Garden Way Publishing, 1975.

Magazines

Countryside, Rt. 1, Box 239, Waterloo, WI 53594.

HORSES
Books
Anderson, Clarence W. *Heads Up, Heels Down.* New York: Macmillan Publishing Co., 1944.

Griffith Rubye, and Griffith, Frank. *Fun of Raising a Colt.* North Hollywood, Calif.: Wilshire Book Co., n.d.

Pittinger, Peggy J. *Back Yard Foal.* North Hollywood, Calif.: Wilshire Book Co., n.d.

Spaulding, Jackie. *The Family Horse: How to Care for, Train and Work with a Horse on the Homestead.* Mayne Island, B.C.: Cloudburst Press, 1979.

Magazines
American Horseman, Countrywide Publications, 257 Park Ave. S., New York, NY 10010.

Horse and Horseman, Charger Productions, 34249 Camino-Capistrano, Capistrano Beach, CA 92624.

Horse and Rider, Rich Publishing, Box 555, Temecula, CA 92390.

Horse Lover's National Magazine, Horse Lover's National, 899 Broadway, Redwood City, CA 94063.

Horse, of Course, Derbyshire Publishing Co., Temple, NH 03084.

DOGS
Books
Complete Dog Book: The Official Publication of the American Kennel Club, 15th ed. New York: Howell Book House, 1975.

Howell Book of Dog Care and Training. New York: Howell Book House, n.d.

Magazines
Dog Fancy, Box 4030, San Clemente, CA 92672.

Dog World, Berner Publishing Co., 10060 W. Roosevelt Rd., Westchester, IL 60153.

CATS

Books

Pond, Grace. *Arco Book of Cats.* New York: Arco Publishing Co., 1969.

Whitney, Leon F. *Complete Book of Cat Care.* Garden City, N.Y.: Double-day & Co., 1953.

Magazines

Cat Fancy, Box 4030, San Clemente, CA 92672.

Cats Magazine, Box 557, Washington, PA 15301.

GENERAL PET MAGAZINES

Animal Lovers, Box 918, New Providence, NJ 07974.

Pet News, 44 Court St., Brooklyn, NY 11201.

Today's Animal Health, Animal Health Foundation, 8338 Rosemead Blvd., Pico Rivera, CA 90660.

ANIMAL HEALTH

Haynes, N. Bruce. *Keeping Livestock Healthy: A Veterinary Guide.* Charlotte, Vt.: Garden Way Publishing, 1978.

Lockwood, Guy C. *Animal Husbandry and Veterinary Care for Self-Sufficient Living.* Phoenix: White Mountain Publishing Co., 1977.

Spaulding, C. E. *A Veterinary Guide for Animal Owners: Cattle, Goats, Sheep, Horses, Pigs, Poultry, Rabbits, Dogs, Cats.* Emmaus, Pa.: Rodale Press, 1976.

Spaulding, Clark, and Spaulding, Jackie. *Dr. Spaulding's Veterinary Answer Book.* Seattle: Madrona Publishers, 1978.

Index

from humane society, 239-242
keeping warm, 91
orphan, 88-92
stimulation of elimination, 89
tube-feeding of, 89-90
vaccinations for, 242
worms in, 92, 96, 242

Q

Quail, 185-86

R

Rabbits, 160-166, 261, 272
  diarrhea in, 164-165
  general care of, 165-166
Rabies
  in wild animals, 121-22, 132,
    144-45, 161, 193-95, 220,
    228-29
  skunks, 193, 233, 235
  vaccine, 96, 149, 233
Raccoons, 143-51, 179, 194, 226-
  27, 270, 274
  chilled, 149
  constipation in, 148-49
  diarrhea in, 147-48
  general care of, 149-50
  orphan, 143-46
  release to wild, 150-51
  vaccinations for, 149
  weaning of, 146-47
Rats, 167-68
Releasing to wild, 217-18
  of bear cubs, 157-59
  of bobcat and cougar kittens,
    139-42
  of coyote, fox, and wolf pups,
    9, 128-29
  of fawns, 111, 116-18

of raccoons and opossums,
  145, 149-50
of squirrels, 162
Rodents
  medium, 160-166
  small, 167-68
Rotenone, 275
  for fleas, 127, 166, 235
  for lice, 81, 188, 235
  for mange, 62
Rumen bacteria, of calves, 48

S

Salt block
  for calves, 54
  for foals, 38
  for kids, 82
Scent, identifying offspring by,
  26, 66-67
Scours. *See* Diarrhea
Scratches, 58, 139, 154, 197
  rabies from, 122, 132, 144
Shelter. *See* Housing
Shock, 59, 68, 92-93, 112, 192,
  215-16, 272
  from bites, 192
  from car accident, 199
Skunks, 193, 233-235, 273
  diet of, 234
  general care of, 234-235
Splint, for broken leg, 112, 201-
  02, 204-05
  simple, 205-06, 209-10
  Thomas, 203, 208
Squirrels, 160-66
  diarrhea in, 164-65
  feeding of, 161-62
  general care of, 165-66
  releasing to wild, 162